WHAT CAN DENTISTRY DO FOR YOU?

A Patient's Guide to Getting that Smile
You Have Always Wanted, Keeping it for a
Lifetime, and Improving Your Health

To Bill and Sheila.

Thanks for your support,

sharing and help over

the years. *Love, Bob*

Robert A. Finkel, DDS, MAGD, FICCMO, FACMS
The Gates at Sugarloaf
1325 Satellite Blvd.
Suite 1304
Suwanee, GA 30024
770-497-9111
www.bobfinkelsmiles.com

WHAT CAN DENTISTRY DO FOR YOU?™

How to contact us:

Robert A. Finkel, DDS, MAGD, FICCMO, FACMS
The Gates at Sugarloaf
1325 Satellite Blvd., Suite 1304
Suwanee, GA 30024

Telephone: 770-497-9111
Fax: 770-623-5594
Web: www.bobfinkelsmiles.com
email: finkeldds@bellsouth.net

Please visit our website and click on our blog!

Acknowledgements

To my wife, Rhonda, my friend, my partner, and my rock,
who has taught me the meaning of love.

To my mom, Iris Finkel,
for her eternal love and support.

To my children, Jeff and Kami,
who have taught me the meaning of family.

To my professional friends and colleagues in Dentistry,
who have shared with me the knowledge
that has made this book possible.

A Note from Dr. Bob Finkel

From a young age, I knew that dentistry was the perfect profession for me. I grew up on Long Island, New York, and always loved science, math, and logic. At age 11, I underwent surgery on my right cheek for removal of a fibro-sarcoma (cancer) and have since felt that people should receive the dental and medical care that will allow them to feel better about themselves.

I attended high school on Long Island and then Union College in Schnectady, New York, where I majored first in physics, and then in computer-chemistry-biology as a combined science major. This allowed me to take my dental school prerequisites while still playing with computers. At this engineering-based school, I was exposed to mechanical engineering concepts which helped fuel my love for dental biomaterials and dental engineering techniques.

Throughout middle school, high school, and college, self-consciousness about my smile and facial surgery helped make me more sympathetic to patients' emotional need to look good and feel confident. My schooling gave me the background to think in engineering terms in designing my dentistry. I was fortunate to have attended Emory University School of Dentistry, considered one of the top five clinical dental schools in the country, and combined my engineering background with dental science. After graduation, I taught part-time at Emory Dental School for one year.

My passions in clinical dental practice are Comprehensive Dental Care, Bio-Engineering and Dental Materials, treatment of Headache and Facial Pain, and improving quality of life through better sleep and Dental Sleep Medicine.

I have practiced for over 33 years in Gwinnett County, Georgia - 10 years in Norcross, 21 years in Duluth, and now in Suwanee. Continuing dental education is a passion for me, and I am honored to have been awarded Fellowship, Mastership, and the Lifetime Learning and Service Award in the Academy of General Dentistry. I enjoy providing comprehensive dental care and working with some of the area's finest dental specialists.

I recognize that properly providing for our patients' long-term oral health needs improves their systemic health and lessens their likelihood of cardiovascular disease, pregnancy problems, Alzheimer's disease, strokes, erectile dysfunction and the like. We are aware of the oral-systemic connection and how proper dental treatment in such areas of periodontal (gum) disease, bite problems, facial pain, and sleep-disordered breathing can contribute to long-term medical health.

I love helping to create smiles, comfort, confidence, and happiness. We enjoy providing conservative treatment to help our patients achieve their long-term goals of dental health, and I cherish our long-term dental and personal relationships. We are honored to have served our patients, their children, and now their children's children.

I am extremely fortunate to be married to my wife, Rhonda, for over 24 years, and to have a son, Jeff, and a daughter, Kami, both of whom I am very proud. Zoe and Ziva, our two dogs, round out our family. Rhonda and I enjoy the north Georgia mountains, hiking, and traveling in Europe.

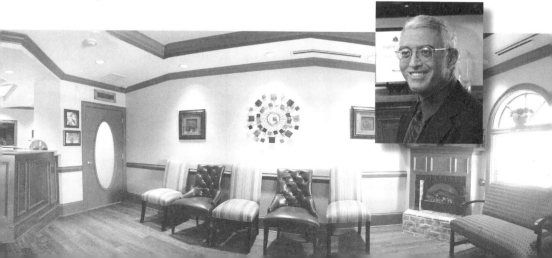

"As a retired practicing dentist of over 35 years, I have been in many, many dental offices and am, of course, very familiar with dental procedures. Dr. Finkel and his staff are by far and away the very best I have ever encountered. Dr. Finkel's attention to detail, excellence, appearance, comfort, and function are unequaled, in my judgment. I have just completed an over two year full mouth reconstruction involving several implants and crowns. I could not be MORE pleased with the results. Just simply outstanding treatment in all respects. His key staff members have been with him for years, which also speaks volumes."

James E. Kelley, DDS

"My teeth have always been a problem for me. It didn't help that I have a big smile. My 20th high school reunion was coming up.

Thank goodness for Dr. Bob and his wonderful staff. I got a new front tooth.

I'm not afraid to smile anymore. I have more confidence in meeting new people. Thanks so much, Dr. Bob!"

Audrey

"I can't say enough to describe Dr. Finkel's outstanding quality of dental care. I will say what I think is equally important is that he truly cares. He cares about each and every individual that he treats, and he cares about each service that he and his staff provide. Excellent dentistry and sincere caring make his practice the perfect place for you and your family."

Dr. Tracy Salyer

Contents

Appendix: Instructions for Patients 234

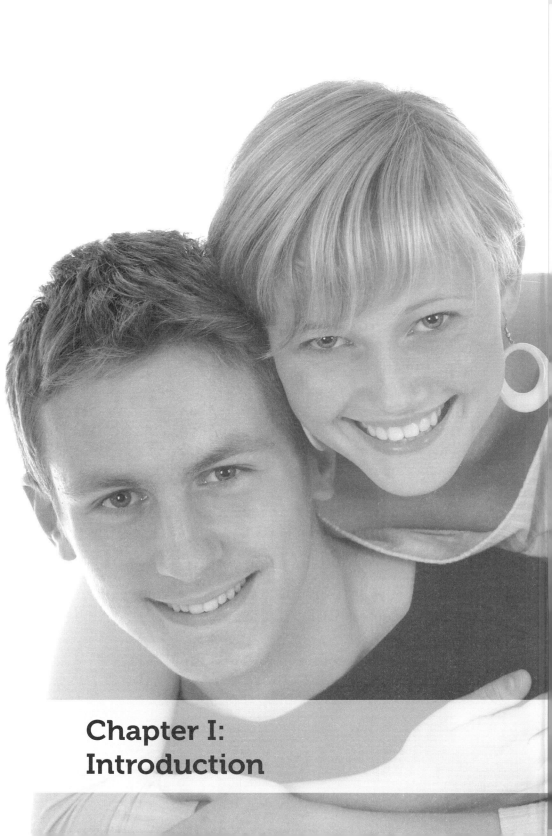

Chapter I:
Introduction

The Value of a Smile

It's hard to overestimate the value of a smile. A smile conveys both warmth and friendship and can serve as an icebreaker in a stressful or unfamiliar situation. People who have unattractive teeth often avoid smiling due to embarrassment and can sometimes suffer from a lack of self-esteem. Fortunately, there is a wide array of dental treatments available that can dramatically improve the appearance of teeth and allow people the ability to smile with confidence.

The most common problems that contribute to an unattractive smile are crooked teeth, as well as teeth that are broken, discolored, loose, or missing. There are dental procedures that can improve each of these situations. If the teeth are crooked, braces can be placed to straighten them. Crooked teeth can also be cosmetically treated with white resin "bonding" and porcelain crowns or facings (veneers) to make them appear straight. Similarly, broken teeth can be restored with white resin bonding or porcelain crowns or veneers. Teeth that are discolored can be whitened with bleaching. Loose and missing teeth can be replaced by a permanent bridge (a series of joined crowns (caps)), implants, or a removable denture. Whatever the dental situation, the appropriate treatment can create a significant improvement in a person's smile and overall dental health.

Having a nice smile can be a great asset in life. Business and social situations are often enhanced by a confident attitude which includes an appealing smile. In my office, I have seen many people who said that their unattractive smile had always made them feel awkward during job interviews. That is why most dentists now realize that they must not only treat the routine and emergency needs of their patients but also consider their cosmetic needs as well. Although it is said that a true smile comes from within, your dentist can certainly improve what everyone sees on the outside.

Choosing Your Dentist

How should you choose your dentist? Price? Special Deal? Reputation? Website? In fact, each and all of these has advantages, so what is the best approach?

Quality dentistry involves a highly educated dentist, up-to-date facilities, a well-trained and well-compensated staff, quality materials and use of quality labs. Mostly, it requires a well-trained and capable dentist. It also involves the dentist and staff taking time to perform your dentistry correctly; giving time to do your dentistry carefully and well.

Quality dentistry also requires that your dentist care enough to put your well-being first and put all the above factors in place so that the patient is priority one. Fees must be high enough to cover the costs of time, quality materials, better labwork, and well-trained staff who aid in your treatment.

In Preferred Provider Plans (PPO'S), know that your insurance company's "Preferred Provider" is not preferred because of quality of care; he or she is preferred because of discounted fees to the insurance company. Avoiding the "PPO Trap" allows you to pick your dental office for caring, commitment, and quality.

So what approach does one take in choosing a dentist? You might check the Academy of General Dentistry for Fellows (FAGD) and Masters (MAGD) in the Academy in your city or area. These are dentists who have spent much time away from family and practice to improve their skills, and in whom you can have confidence and trust.

Also, check out other legitimate academies in the dental field for dentists with additional training in those fields. A Fellow in the International College of Cranomandibular Orthopedics (FICCMO) is a dentist with greater training in treatment of facial pain, TM joint problems, and bite mal-alignments. Look for academies that are older, larger, and more recognized, so you can feel good about your choice of dentist.

Your previous dentist may have knowledge of a qualified, credentialed dentist in your new area. If you have friends that work in a dental lab or dental specialist's office, ask them whose dental work is most indicative of quality, caring, and skill among the dentists whose work they see.

"Best Dentist" awards should be based on recognition by peers and dental specialists, who can judge quality and skill, and may help steer you to a qualified, caring dentist.

Once you choose a dentist or narrow down your choices, what is next? You should feel free to schedule a non-treatment visit to the office to meet the staff, tour the office, and see if the practice is right for you.

If testimonials on a dental office website are true, the office should be able to get one or more of the happy patients to speak with you by phone regarding desired treatment similar to theirs. Verifiable before and after stories and photos should be available to you.

Remember that dental full-mouth rehabilitation will likely cost the same

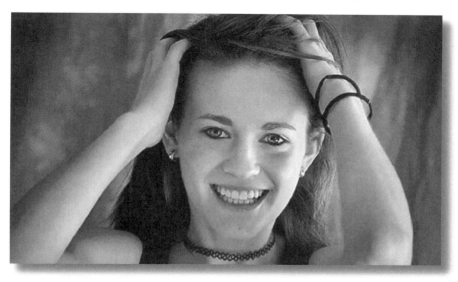

as a new car. It is a large investment in time, money, and trust. You must choose your dentist with greater care than you might choose the type and cost of a new car. You want to choose your dentist as someone you trust to recommend your best care, perform it properly, and to be available and responsive to you as time goes on.

What Sets Us Apart

We are recognized in the community for creating smiles with conservative, long-lasting, techniques.

Many of our patients have trusted us to care for them, their children, and their grandchildren for over 30 years.

Local dental laboratories consider our dentistry to be of the highest quality, precision, and longevity.

We offer a variety of in-office dental services so patients don't need to run from office to office to complete their dental care. Restorative dentistry, endodontics, periodontics, headache therapy, dental sleep therapy and oral surgery may be required to complete a case and may be provided all in our office.

We are able to improve your smile and re-balance your bite easily and comfortably.

We have completed thousands of hours of continuing dental education so you can receive the best care.

We have a good team approach to your dental care and coordinate with the finest dental specialists in the area to provide your treatment.

We treat many local physicians and dentists.

We have authored two books, and lecture to physicians and other dentists on treatment for headache, facial pain, and sleep problems.

We strive to make premium dentistry affordable for you.

We are involved in our local county Executive Roundtable, support various community causes, and strongly support the Wounded Warrior Project for our wounded veterans and the Atlanta Community Food Bank.

We have an incredible caring, dedicated, and highly trained dental staff.

What to Expect in Your Dental Office

Now that you have picked your dentist, what should you expect from him or her, the office, and the dental staff?

Firstly, respect for your time, money, values, and uniqueness as a person. There is no "one-size-fits-all" style of dentistry. You may want efficient, no-nonsense dental visits with good quality, but no social amenities. You may want Spa-style dentistry in which each visit is a pampering experience, and you are happy to allocate the time and money for that. Each is a valid choice.

You may desire full-mouth rehabilitation to the level and cost of a new car (What level? Which car?). You may want maintenance of your existing dentistry with no major changes.

You may desire a full smile make-over with a Hollywood dazzle, or you may be fine with your smile but desire maximum functionality and durability. Cost may be a major consideration, a minor detail, or, value-per-dollar, somewhere in-between.

Your goals:

Whatever your goals, your dentist and dental staff should listen to you, discern your goals and values, and present options that are workable for you. Your dentist's goal should be to remain your dentist for as long as he or she is in practice. Your dentist should ask for and receive your permission to look in your mouth, inform you of what he or she sees, and recommend to you what he would recommend to a member of his or her family. Out of what your dentist recommends in treatment, you should feel free to accept all of it, none of it, or some of it without hurting his or her (the dentist's) feelings.

When you walk out of the dental office door, you should have the information you need to make an informed decision on your own behalf. You may be able to afford your desired treatment immediately, over time, or never; but you should understand all of your options and be able to make an informed choice.

Your dentist should passionately recommend what he or she feels is best for you, actively discourage less-healthy options, and always be your advocate. Remember, as dentists, we work for you; we should be present as a coach, facilitator, and provider of service but never as a salesman and never as one who dictates what treatment you choose.

Your health:

What should your dentist look for?

In the past, dentists were expected to look for decay (cavities) and gum disease (periodontitis). They were expected to handle bite problems and replace missing teeth.

We now more fully understand the connection between oral problems, ongoing tooth loss, headache, facial pain, and many systemic health issues.

Your Dentist Should Check For:

1. Decay (cavities) and chemical erosion of the teeth

2. Broken teeth or damage from aggressive tooth brushing

3. Gum disease (periodontitis) or gum recession

4. Changes in the appearance of oral tissues (possible cancer)

5. Orthodontic (tooth & jaw alignment) problems

6. Endodontic (root canal) problems

7. Bite (occlusal) problems

8. Joint and jaw ("TMJ" or "TMD") problems

9. Esthetic problems (color, shape, size, position, alignment) of teeth

10. Disturbances in function and comfort

11. Any other risks to health of the teeth, gum, mouth, joints, or muscles

X-rays (radiographs) should be taken to check for:

1. Decay (cavities)

2. Bone loss

3. Cysts, tumors, cancers, or impacted teeth

4. Abcesses

5. Bone problems of the upper or lower jaw

6. Joint changes

7. Changes in normal bone, joints or soft tissue

8. Sinus problems

9. Any other abnormalities of the jaws or face

Clinical Examinations May Involve:

1. Special gum probes: simple (manual) or computerized

2. Jaw tracking to ensure normal jaw joint and muscle movement

3. Muscle function testing

4. Vitality (tooth nerve health) tests

5. Special cavity tests with lasers and/or computers

6. Saliva tests for cancer, Human Papilloma (cancer-associated) Virus; chemical tests for periodontal damaging bacteria; genetic tests for periodontal disease susceptibility; tests for acid-buffering (cavity-neutralizing) factors, diabetes, and other health problems

7. Cancer screening with optical devices, special lights, chemicals and saliva-tests

The dentist should also check for any other obvious problems that create risk to health of the teeth, gums and jaw structures. Technology is continually giving us new ways to use saliva-testing to check for systemic (body) health issues or medical diseases. Our abilities to test for general health problems using saliva will continue to expand and grow as time goes on.

You should expect your dentist to explore your choices, dental goals and values, and perform a thorough examination of your current oral and dental situation. Past dental experiences and treatments should be reviewed, as well as general health conditions. The dentist should also look for factors such as dry mouth (xerostomia), bruxism (grinding), oral habits, damaging foods or drinks, consumption of acid beverages, and health problems (such as G.E.R.D. or bulimia) which can damage teeth.

Once the examination is completed, the data gathered, and problems identified, the dentist should provide treatment options to coincide with your personal values and goals. Now your choices begin, and you choose which option(s) align with your goals and resources. It is better to work on long-term treatment goals, even if handled over time, than to choose less comprehensive treatment, simply because it is faster and/or cheaper. If your dental goals exceed your current resources, ask your dentist how that treatment can be staged over time to accommodate your financial and personal needs.

In a modern, up-to-date dental office, you should be given choices, you should have access to the types of dentistry that best serve you, and your dentist should explore the connections between systemic (medical) health and oral (dental) health. In later chapters, we will review the effects of periodontal disease on the body and the ways in which periodontal disease can initiate or worsen general medical issues. We will also present a white paper for you and your physician regarding this medical/dental connection. For now, please understand that your dentist should be a partner with your physician in maintaining your overall health and that here are some of the areas for partnership:

Chronic bad breath that won't go away can be a sign of gum disease and active infection with dozens of potentially harmful bacteria which are often found in the thickened and diseased blood vessels of the heart. If the bad breath that won't go away isn't caused by gum disease, then other body malfunctions may be detected. For example, your breath will smell different if you have uncontrolled diabetes.

Perhaps, upon examination, your dentist finds significant dental decay and general breakdown of your teeth. You are bewildered because you know that you eat well and take good general care of your teeth. Later, with more evaluation, you find that you were right all along. But you didn't know you had GERD, Gastro-Esophageal Reflux Disease, with high acidity literally eating away your teeth. If you didn't know this you could have just given up and blamed it on bad genetics. Knowing the real reason, you can control your gastric reflux and keep your teeth and gums healthy. Many medications also cause dry-mouth, and too little saliva can greatly increase tooth decay.

Perhaps, you notice your teeth are worn and they are getting worse. You often wake up with headaches and feel moody and grumpy during the day even though you get enough sleep. This could have easily gone undetected. An expert dentist would have questioned you about your sleep and breathing because when you experience excessive wear of your teeth, you often have sleep-disordered breathing or Obstructive Sleep Apnea (OSA), which can be life threatening!

Who knew of such things? Most people just don't make the connection.

Part of modern dental practice includes regular care to check the gums, teeth, and mouth for problems before they become larger and more expensive, and looking for oral signs of systemic health problems to refer you to your MD for evaluation.

Periodontal (gum) infection is caused by the bacteria around the teeth invading deeper gum pockets and setting up inflammatory processes by which the body tries to rid itself of the bacteria and infected teeth. All forms of periodontal disease (Periodontitis), from mild to extremely destructive, cause the body's defense systems to produce many chemicals ("inflammatory mediators") called cytokines, which act as messengers telling the body that infection is present and that the body needs to ramp up its ability to fight the infection.

These cytokines instruct the body as to where and how to defend itself and fight the infection. They also signal the liver to produce C-Reactive Protein (CRP) as an indicator of ongoing defense. CRP is an indicator of ongoing infection/damage, but also seems to be a cause of additional damage to the body, far from the original site of infection. So CRP levels indicate not only the presence of destructive body processes, but also, seemingly, are a cause of additional damage.

CRP is heavily studied for its roles as both indicator and cause of health problems, but research already indicates that periodontal infection and high CRP levels are associated with:

1. Heart disease, coronary artery disease, heart attacks, and stroke

2. High cholesterol and high blood pressure

3. Diabetes and obesity (associated with higher blood levels of HgA1C [indicator of blood sugar levels]), Metabolic Syndrome

4. Gestational (pregnancy) diabetes

5. Preterm delivery and gestational high blood pressure

6. Preterm birth problems for the infant such as low birth weight, brain problems, cardiac (heart) problems, eye problems, and respiratory (breathing) problems [related to the cytokines produced by the mother in response to gum infection]

7. Cancer

8. Osteoporosis

9. HIV reactivation in patients with latent HIV infection, leading to AIDS

10. Gastric (stomach) ulcers

11. Arthritis

What is the bottom line? It is that oral bacteria cause periodontal disease (periodontitis) resulting in gum infections and inflammation, then release of cytokines and production of C-Reactive Protein (CRP), and initiation or worsening of systemic disease. Properly treating periodontal disease reduces the bacterial infection, the body's inflammatory load, and the production of CRP. These lower levels of CRP are associated with lower risk of the above-listed conditions.

You should choose a dental office in which these medical/dental connections are understood and in which your dentist can be in partnership with you and your physician for your better health.

Comprehensive Dental Care

What is comprehensive dental care? It is the combination of proper examination, diagnosis, treatment planning, and treatment, so that the dentistry you receive is exactly what you need and is done well. It is complete care, so that you may experience all areas of dentistry, not just the limited areas of dentistry that your dentist may be familiar with. You want the dentistry that will allow you to maintain dental youth and not slide into dental old age. Your goal should be to stay as dentally young as possible.

You should plan for restoration of the teeth that you have, replacement of the missing ones, maintenance of your dental restorations, comfort of your dental restorations, and long-term function of the dentistry you have invested in. You should not continually experience loss of teeth and you should be happy with your smile, the overall look of your teeth, your ability to chew, your comfort, and your confidence when facing other people. The longer you live, the longer you need to maintain your smile and your dental health; if you are in need of advanced dentistry, then you should feel confident that any dentistry you have performed is geared to last you as long as possible.

Proper dentistry requires a complete dental examination. Your dentist should take x-rays, photographs, and perform a full exam with study models, bite records, and gum charting as needed to assess your dental health. In complex cases, models, bite records, and other diagnostic aids are often necessary as part of your exam. In diagnosis, your dentist should be evaluating your teeth for strength, decay, (what most people call cavities), periodontal disease, bite problems, jaw problems, muscle problems, and cancer-related problems. Anything out of the ordinary should be identified by your dentist at the exam as part of his findings. The diagnosis may involve more than one visit and, if your dentistry is complicated, then you should allow your dentist sufficient time to ensure that he can determine what you really need.

So your dentist should, among other things, check for decay (cavities) and for periodontal (gum) disease. The dentist should check for stress and wear on your teeth and possibly a mis-matched bite that no longer supports your teeth, your joints, and your muscles. The dentist should also look for systemic problems such as GERD, diabetes, heart disease, history of stroke, and other systemic diseases aggravated by dental problems.

Once your dentist has identified your dental problems, he or she should then provide you with options for fixing those problems and restoring your mouth to optimum health. You might need treatment for bite problems, headaches, TMJ pain, cavities, gum disease, joint problems, or muscle problems. Your dentist should be able to provide you with treatment in the areas of gum therapy, fillings, crowns, root canals, dentures, bridges, implants, biopsies, and anything else that aids in (re-) building the smile you have always wanted. Your dentist should either provide these services directly or work with a team of specialists that can provide these treatments at the highest level.

An important treatment concept should be over-engineering of the dentistry you receive. The dentistry should not be performed just to the level that you accept and will pay for it, but should be done to the level that the dentist would want for a member of his own family or himself, and should always be designed to last as long as possible. Follow-up care should also be provided; cleanings, fluoride trays, and night guards to help protect the dentistry that was done, and other specialized care such as dry mouth care, or more frequent cleanings to avoid the recurrence of gum disease or at least keep it at bay. Certain medications are now also used to help keep gum disease under control, and this may be part of your ongoing care. Your dentist should also be able to provide you with sedation for complex dental appointments and other amenities that help make your dental visits more comfortable.

In summary, comprehensive care dentistry is a program of examination, diagnosis, treatment planning, and treatment so that you receive the greatest possible options for your dental treatment. Also, whatever dental treatment you receive is rendered at the highest level in a way that is over-engineered, to last as long as possible for you, and that follow-up care helps maintain your dentistry as long as possible.

One final note in the arena of comprehensive dentistry: this book has a section on the Oral-Systemic connection, or how conditions in the body are affected by conditions in the mouth. There are many areas of systemic health that can be optimized by maximizing your dental health. If you take a look at that section, you will notice that bite problems can cause headaches, facial pain, and joint and muscle problems. Periodontal (gum) infections can aggravate conditions leading to cardiovascular disease, stroke, and kidney disease. Sleep problems can aggravate many of the same systemic problems, including aggravating Metabolic Syndrome, heart disease, kidney disease, stroke, and high blood pressure. Comprehensive dental care involves proper dentistry as well as proper management of those oral conditions that affect your systemic health and overall well-being. A well-informed dentist should guide you to maximum health in all the areas of the mouth and body that are interrelated.

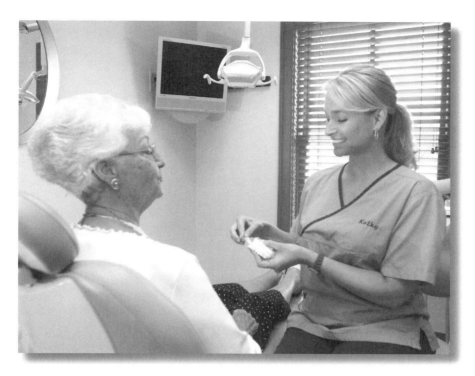

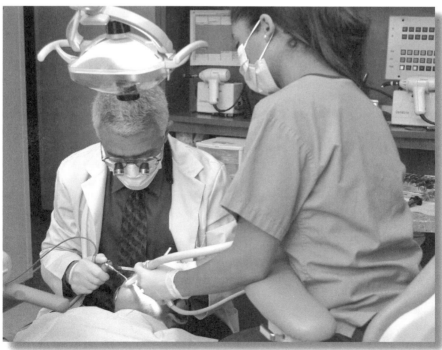

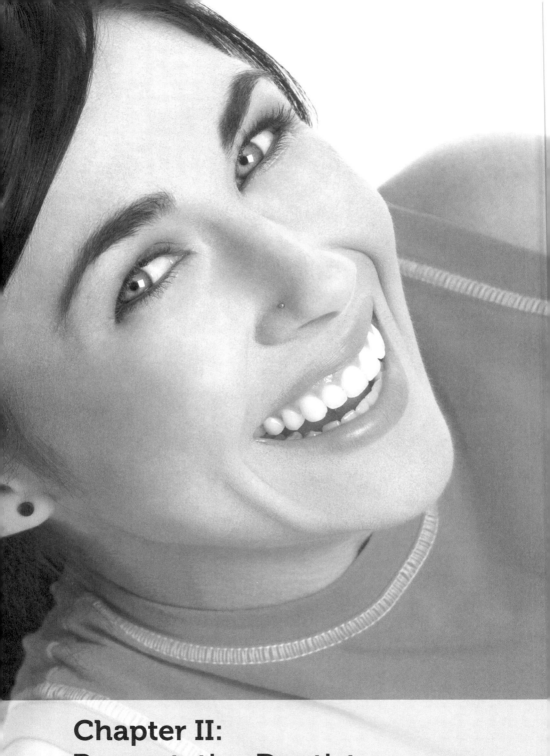

Chapter II:
Preventative Dentistry

Preventative Dental Care

We recommend regular dental care to keep your smile healthy and to keep little problems from becoming bigger problems. Each individual's situation is unique and different, but our general recommendations are:

Comprehensive New Patient Exam
— Recommended every 3 years

Dental Cleaning with Periodic Exam
— Recommended every 3 to 6 months
— Recommended every 3 months for patients with a history of or active periodontal disease (keeps down bacteria count on teeth and in the gums)

Bitewing X-rays (cavity detecting x-rays)
— Recommended once per year or as indicated

Panoramic X-ray (scanning x-ray)
— Recommended every 3 to 5 years

Oral Cancer Screening using the Velscope
— Recommended yearly

Periodontal Screening
— Evaluating the gums and bone supporting the teeth
— At least twice yearly

Cosmetic Evaluation
— For smile factors
— As desired

Fluoride Treatment
— Shown to be beneficial for children and adults
— At cleanings and/or at home daily

Sealants
— What are <u>sealants</u>? A dental sealant is a plastic material that is applied to the chewing surface of a tooth. It acts as a barrier, protecting enamel by sealing out plaque and food. The teeth are cleaned and prepared and the sealant bonded on the tooth enamel which then hardens on the tooth. Sealants are usually clear or white and not visible when you talk or smile. They can help prevent decay and save money in the future on restorative procedures, and should be applied to the teeth within six months of the teeth erupting into the mouth.

Dry Mouth (Xerostomia) and Aggressive Cavities (Decay)

Many people produce less saliva as they grow older. This decrease can also be caused by many common medications, chemotherapy, and some radiation therapies for cancer. Saliva is the great protector of your teeth and gums. Anything that decreases saliva production becomes a threat to your oral health. Also, many individuals have more aggressive cavities (decay), greater susceptibility to cavities, or the presence of more aggressive decay-causing bacteria in their mouth because of neglected home care.

Saliva's Benefits

Like a well- known comedian's lament, saliva just doesn't get any respect. You probably take it for granted, never realizing the important role it plays in keeping your mouth and teeth healthy.

Saliva helps prevent tooth decay and gum disease by removing food debris from the mouth and neutralizing bacterial acids. Because it contains the same minerals found in tooth enamel (calcium and phosphate), saliva works with fluoride to "repair" or "heal" tooth enamel whenever early cavities begin to form.

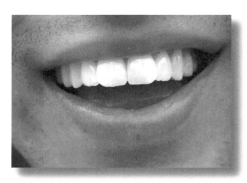

Unfortunately, one in seven adults suffers from impaired salivary function, a condition known as "dry mouth." Dry mouth, or xerostomia, can be a symptom of aging or a side effect of more than 430 different medications (including antidepressants, antihypertensives, and antihistamines). It can also result from radiation therapy to salivary glands.

If you suffer from "dry mouth," talk to a dental professional. Dental professionals can often provide helpful dietary guidelines for their patients. In addition, they can prescribe an artificial saliva product to help supplement normal salivary flow.

Treatment for Dry Mouth (Xerostomia) and Aggressive Cavities (Decay)

Note: 1. Saliva washes acid from plaque/bacteria off the teeth. Saliva also buffers (neutralizes) these acids.
2. Calcium and phosphate salts in saliva remineralize (rebuild) the tooth enamel.
3. Too little saliva results in extreme decay (cavities) and severe periodontial (gum) disease.
4. Fluoride helps saliva protect enamel; it builds stronger (more acid-resistant) enamel and inhibits bacteria.
5. Age, medications, and conditions like diabetes may cause decreased salivation and dry mouth (xerostomia).
6. Age, dry mouth, and acidic drinks (eg. sodas) can initiate root decay and tooth loss.

1. Practice meticulous homecare – brush, floss, fluoride use, plus tongue scraper!! Floss, then brush (not too forcefully), starting at a different position in the mouth (teeth) each time. Thoroughly clean/scrape the tongue as far back as possible. Have 3-month cleanings. Ideally use Peridex (chlorhexidine) rinse for 30 seconds twice daily for two weeks prior to each 3-month cleaning.

2. Use high-level fluoride toothpaste plus fluoride rinse. Spit out; do not rinse. The most effective method is to use mouth trays with fluoride gel four minutes per day. Use while showering, dressing, or some other regular daily activity. 3-month fluoride varnish treatments are also beneficial.

3. Use MI paste to remineralize the teeth. Brush the teeth with MI paste. Do not rinse or spit. You can use trays on teeth for five minutes. Remove trays and spit. Do not rinse. Alternate high-level fluoride therapy for one month, then MI paste for one month. **Do not use MI paste if dairy-allergic.**

4. Drink plenty of water (large container sipped throughout the day) and/or suck on ice chips.

5. Use sugarless gum, candies, snacks with Xylitol (no citric acid) to stimulate saliva and inhibit oral bacteria. Chew Xylitol-based gum, such as Biotene, for at least three minutes five times daily.

6. Use salivary substitutes (Salivart, Xerolube, Biotene, Oasis, etc.). Rinse/swish/use small spray bottle frequently. Biotene and Oasis have good lines of rinse, oral gel, and xylitol-based gum.

7. Use a powered toothbrush to keep mouth cleaner (eg., Sonicare, Oral B or Ultreo).

8. Use Salistat tablets or other xylitol-based tablets as needed, to stimulate salivary flow.

9. Avoid carbonated drinks (sodas) and sports/energy drinks. All such drinks are extremely acidic and damaging. Acidity is measured by pH. The lower the pH number the more acidic and damaging. A pH of 6.5 dissolves dentin (root). A pH of 5.5 dissolves enamel. Carbonated drinks (sodas) such as Gatorade and Red Bull have a pH

of 3+, very damaging! Drink sodas quickly, never sip slowly. Fruit juices must be calcium-fortified to minimize tooth damage.

10. Limit snacks (especially carbs and sugars) to 3 times daily and avoid drinks described in #9. After snacks and drinks, rinse teeth with water. If the drinks/snacks are acidic, rinse with an antacid liquid. Do not brush the now–weakened enamel. Wait 1 hour to brush. Brush gently, always beginning the tooth brushing in a different location.

11. Use an anti-microbial (germ-killing) rinse such as Peridex-type or Crest Pro-Health Rinse two to three times daily.

12. Be aware of your medications that might cause dry mouth. Ask your doctor about changing to a similar medication with fewer dry-mouth effects. Ask for Cevimeline or a similar medication to stimulate saliva production.

13. Know that this may be a long-term problem, requiring a long-term commitment on your part.

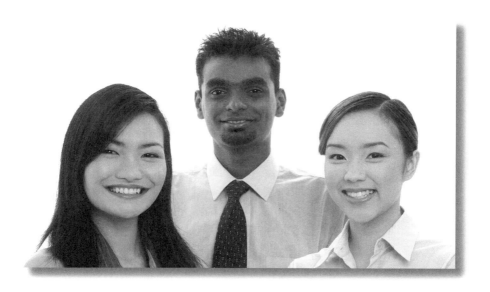

Fluorides

Most of us have heard that fluoride is good for our teeth without any real explanation as to how and why. Here is what you might want to know about fluoride and teeth.

What is Fluoride?

Fluoride is a form of the chemical element Fluorine which, when chemically incorporated into tooth structure, makes the tooth structure stronger and more decay-resistant. When the teeth are developing in the jaws, not yet erupted into the mouth, they are actually still in the body and their chemical composition can be modified by the body, dependent upon what nutrients (such as fluoride) are available in the diet. Once the teeth have erupted in the mouth (technically out of the body), the tooth surfaces are most affected by what occurs in the mouth immediately around them. Bacteria can now colonize (stick to) the teeth and produce chemicals, including acids, which attack and eat away at the enamel (harder, tougher) and dentin (softer, more easily damaged) surfaces of the teeth.

What about acids? The tooth, the whole tooth, and nothing but the tooth:

Acids from sodas, energy drinks, sports drinks, and acidic fruit juices can also directly attack the tooth surfaces, as well as providing vast amounts of sugar and other carbohydrates that the dental bacteria convert into acids to additionally attack the teeth. The acids and the sugar also greatly increase the ability of these acid-producing bacteria to grow.

Sugar + acid + bad bacteria → More bad bacteria →

More acids → More Decay

As more acid is produced on the teeth, the tooth surfaces become more acidic (lower pH), and at a certain level of acidity (lowered pH), the acids dissolve the calcium and phosphate mineral structure out of the teeth.

Minerals are continually moving out of the tooth surface into the saliva (demineralization) and back from the saliva into the tooth surface (remineralization) in an equilibrium that keeps the tooth surface intact. Above a critical level of acidity (critically lowered pH), the tooth structure is more dissolved (demineralization). Above this critical pH (lower acid), the minerals of the tooth surface move back in (remineralization) and are in equilibrium; they move in and out of the tooth surface at about the same rate and the tooth surface stays whole. With higher acid levels, minerals move out of the tooth surface (decay, cavities); with lower acid levels, the tooth stays undamaged.

To dissolve the (tougher) enamel requires a moderate amount of acid (critical pH); to dissolve the (weaker) dentin takes less acid, and is more easily accomplished.

So how do Fluorides help?

1. Fluoride inhibits tooth demineralization by shifting the chemical equilibrium so more acid is required to dissolve minerals out of the tooth structure.

2. Fluoride encourages remineralization of the tooth by the calcium and phosphate salts in saliva, shifting the chemical equilibrium so they move back into the tooth.

3. Fluoride makes the remineralized tooth structure (enamel and dentin) more stable and more resistant to acid attack and acid erosion.

4. Fluoride decreases tooth sensitivity.

5. Fluoride inhibits the bacterial enzyme systems that cause tooth damage.

6. Fluoride is bacteriocidal against (kills) many damaging oral bacteria.

7. Fluoride decreases the ability of the bad bacteria to stick to the teeth.

8. Fluorides can remain on and in the tooth surface for extended periods of time to provide on-going protection.

9. Fluorides can help other tooth remineralization technologies, such as Recaldent, MI paste, and Xylitol, work more effectively.

How do we get this fluoride protection?

Fluoride in the water supply helps incorporate fluoride into the tooth structure as it is being formed, for long-term cavity protection. Studies have shown it to protect against some forms of cancer. Too high a level in the water supply can cause teeth to have white spots ("fluorosis") – often imparting a very pretty effect to the teeth. Too low a level provides little dental protection. Perhaps some harmless white spots, with fluoride in the water, are better than many dark spots (cavities, decay) resulting from no fluoride protection.

Fluorides come in many forms; gels, toothpastes, rinses, and creams. They can be applied in many ways; as toothpaste, in daily-use trays, as varnishes to paint on teeth, as varnishes to be light-cured onto teeth, or incorporated into dental restorative materials. Whatever the form and method of application, topical (surface-applied) fluoride becomes attached to the surface of the tooth (adsorbed) and incorporated into the surface structure to provide the protections listed above.

Consuming vast amounts of anything (like swallowing lots of fluoride gel or eating a whole tube of toothpaste) can cause illness, so care should always be taken to avoid this. We don't let our kids eat other chemicals; fluoride gel and toothpaste should receive the same consideration.

What about Xerostomia ("Dry Mouth") and Fluoride?

Xerostomia ("Dry Mouth") is a condition in which the patient produces too little saliva. It is often not recognized by the patient until saliva production has decreased by 70%. Without enough saliva to remove and buffer mouth acids, damage to the teeth can occur with a 40% loss of saliva, so oral damage is often occurring without the patient recognizing the problem of too little saliva production.

Xerostomia has many possible causes. It may be caused by Sjogren's Syndrome of dry eyes, dry mouth, and dryness of other delicate body membranes, or it may be a side effect of other auto-immune diseases such as rheumatoid arthritis. It may be the result of many drugs such as anti-depresssants, sedatives, pain medications, and antihistamines. Xerostomia may also be the result of diabetes, chemotherapy, or radiation therapy for cancer. Whatever the cause, dry mouth results in the presence of less saliva and more acid-damage of the teeth.

Fluoride treatment is often combined with other treatments to help give protection where there is not enough saliva to wash acids off the teeth and to buffer (neutralize) the acids. It is usually combined with other protective strategies. Please see our section (p. 32) on Xerostomia (Dry Mouth) and Aggressive Cavities Treatment.

So; final answer?

Fluoride can help protect the teeth from too much acid, too much sugar, and too little saliva. Minimal dental problems require minimal use of fluoride; greater dental problems (decay and periodontal disease) require greater use of fluoride for protection. We will be happy to discuss if and how fluoride treatment can be of benefit to you.

Fluoride Research

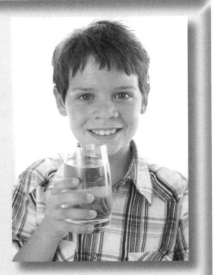

About 55% of Americans drink fluoridated water supplied by their communities. But what about the 45% that do not?

A recent study's preliminary results indicate that daily fluoride tablets, combined with weekly fluoride rinses, work best at fighting cavities in communities where water fluoridation is not adequate.

Researchers compared the amount of tooth decay in children receiving weekly fluoride rinses, daily fluoride tablets, or both procedures combined. Those children who received the combined fluoride treatment experienced almost a third less tooth decay than children who merely rinsed with the fluoride solution.

Although the children who received fluoride tablets had more tooth decay than those who received the combined fluoride treatment, the differences between the two groups were not significant.

These findings indicate that for communities without fluoridated water supplies, the fluoride tablet alone is the most cost-effective strategy for preventing cavities in children.

This procedure is also easier than the combined fluoride rinse and tablet treatment.

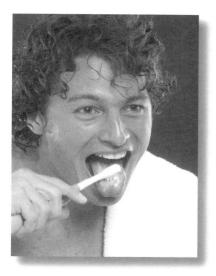

Stick Out Your Tongue to Bad Breath

Proper oral hygiene should include brushing teeth, gums, and, yes, the tongue. Regular tongue brushing for adults with healthy gums can greatly improve breath quality, according to researchers at Case Western Reserve University in Cleveland, Ohio.

The tongue, which occupies one-third of the mouth, provides a warm, moist breeding ground for bacteria. Bacteria counts can increase tenfold after only one week without brushing the tongue.

If you have healthy teeth and gums, tongue brushing or tongue scraping can go a long way to improve your mouth odor. But if you have another notorious cause of bad breath, such as gum disease, you need to give us a call.

In one study involving 30 adults with healthy teeth and gums, the group was divided into two sub-groups, each employing a different tongue-cleansing method. The first group used a toothbrush, and the second group used a tongue scraper— a thin plastic or metal strip that can be bent into a U-shape. Those who used the tongue scrapers enjoyed the greatest improvement in breath, although tongue brushers also had significantly better breath. The second study involving 18 adults suffering from gum disease, concluded that tongue brushing alone did not reduce bad breath. Mouth odor caused by gum disease won't go away with brushing. The only way to treat bad breath in such cases is by treating the gum disease first. If bad breath is a concern for you, call us for a breath analysis and treatment.

Icon: No-Drill Dental Work

Icon is a new way your dentist can stop the progression of an early cavity before it needs to be treated using a needle or drill. This breakthrough treatment preserves healthy tooth structure, prolonging the life expectancy of natural teeth and is completed in just one visit.

Introduced by DMG America in September 2009, Icon® uses microinvasive technology to fill and reinforce demineralized enamel without drilling, anesthesia, or sacrificing healthy tooth structure. Icon, which stands for Infiltration Concept, is a true breakthrough in restorative dentistry indicated for the treatment of white spot lesions and incipient decay that has progressed up to the first third of dentin. Icon® enables dentists to treat incipient lesions upon discovery, effectively removing white spots and arresting the progression of early carious lesions. It works by capillary action and is light cured to harden the resin after placement. Previously, it was necessary for dental professionals to "wait and watch" early caries until they were big enough to justify drilling and filling, and they had only more invasive options for treating discoloration such as white spot lesions that could not be eliminated by tooth whitening.

For more information visit www.drilling-no-thanks.com.

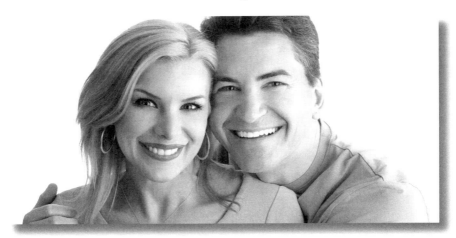

Mouthguards: Playing it Safe!

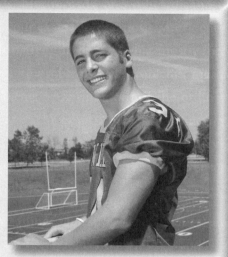

When it comes to sports, don't underestimate the value of a mouth guard.

A mouthguard should be worn during most sport activities. Mouthguards help prevent tooth loss and damage and bruising of lips and cheeks.

Of all the injuries documented in a study of junior and senior high school football, baseball, and basketball players, 40% occurred during basketball and baseball games or practice.

Mouthguards are sold in sports stores or drugstores and are available in three sizes. A custom fitted mouthguard made for players will provide more reliable protection. The parents of young athletes should consider this option. Ask us about it!

"For many years, my smile was becoming worse as time went by. I had become BILLY BOB. Then, Dr. Bob fixed my smile. Now I can smile with confidence."

Marty

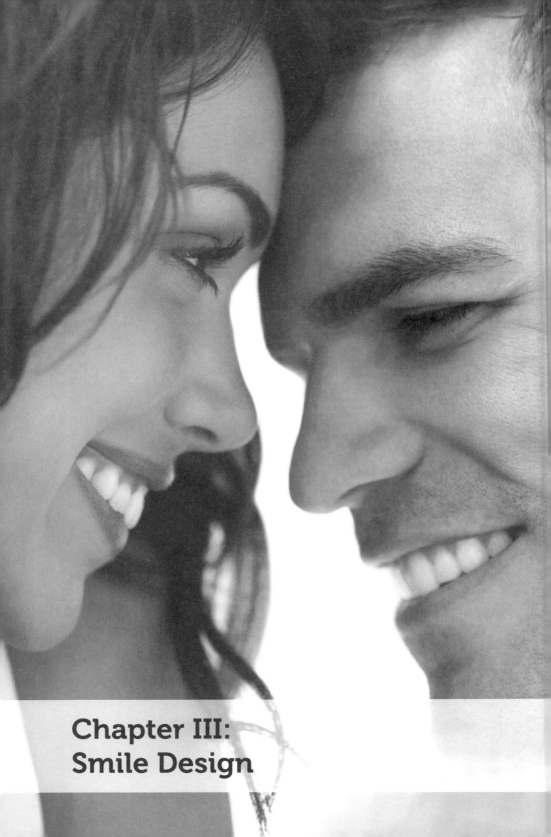

Chapter III:
Smile Design

Smile Design

Smile design is the process of analyzing the smile you have and what needs to be done to give you the smile you want. Some of the factors we analyze are tooth color, shape, size, angle, and spacing. We also analyze how the teeth fit in the lips and the face while properly supporting the lips, cheeks and face. Smile design also includes proper phonetics (speech), bite support, function, general health and overall pleasing appearance. All of these esthetic, biomechanical, and functional factors must be taken into account when designing your new individualized smile.

Cosmetic Contouring (Shaping)

If your front teeth are healthy and sound, but somewhat ragged and chipped, we can often revitalize your smile with some smoothing, rounding, and shaping of the edges. Done in a gentle and conservative fashion, this is often the easiest way to improve the appearance of your teeth. If combined with bleaching (whitening) of the teeth and possibly some minor bonding, we can often give your smile a much more youthful look with a minimum of cost, time, and bother.

Teeth Whitening

Professional tooth whitening is a bleaching process that lightens discolored teeth. There are many causes for discolored teeth. The most common is age and consumption of staining substances (coffee, tea, soft drinks, and tobacco), trauma, and old restorations. Most people can benefit from tooth whitening; the degree of whitening will vary from patient to patient. Tooth whitening is very safe when performed under the supervision of a dentist.

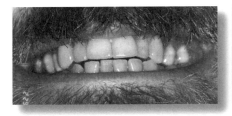 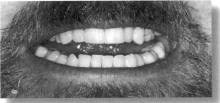

What is the Process of bleaching?

Impressions of your upper and lower teeth will be taken. This will allow us to make a custom fitting whitening tray. You will be given whitening gel and specific instructions on how to use the gel and how often. We will continue to see you every 2-3 weeks until you reach your desired shade. The results are safer, gentler, and more long-lasting than those of strips or in-office "power" bleaching.

Tooth Colored Fillings

If you dislike the look of your dark silver fillings, or you want the strength that bonded tooth-colored fillings can give your teeth, we can help. Replacing any old dark, defective fillings with the newer composite bonded fillings can help make your teeth stronger and your smile more attractive. The newer bonded fillings cost a little more and take a little longer to place, but are a definite plus if you value your smile.

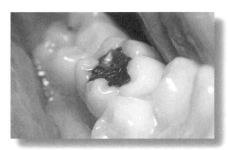 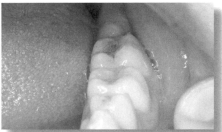

Bonding and Veneers

We can beautify your smile in a conservative manner with composite bonding and porcelain veneers. Composite bonding is done directly on the teeth, sculpting tooth-colored bonding material onto the teeth to correct spaces, enamel defects, and discolorations. The material is then cured (solidified), adjusted, and polished.

Porcelain veneers, created on a model (impression) of your prepared teeth, are thin porcelain shells which are then bonded to your teeth for a more fabulous smile.

Composite bonding is usually more conservative of tooth structure and more economical. Porcelain veneers are more solid and durable, but more costly. Either or both can help give you the smile of your dreams.

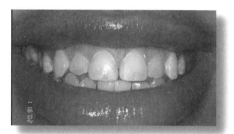 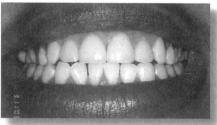

Refer to the chapter on Bonding (p. 130) and the chapter on Veneers (p. 134) for further information.

"Dr. Finkel and his staff are professionals, and Dr. Finkel in particular is very caring and a perfectionist. He likes to make sure that everything is perfect.

"I also like it that Dr. Finkel calls his patients in the evening, to make sure that we are doing okay, painwise.

"I came to see Dr. Finkel for bleaching my teeth and for the cleaning. They are excellent."

Constance

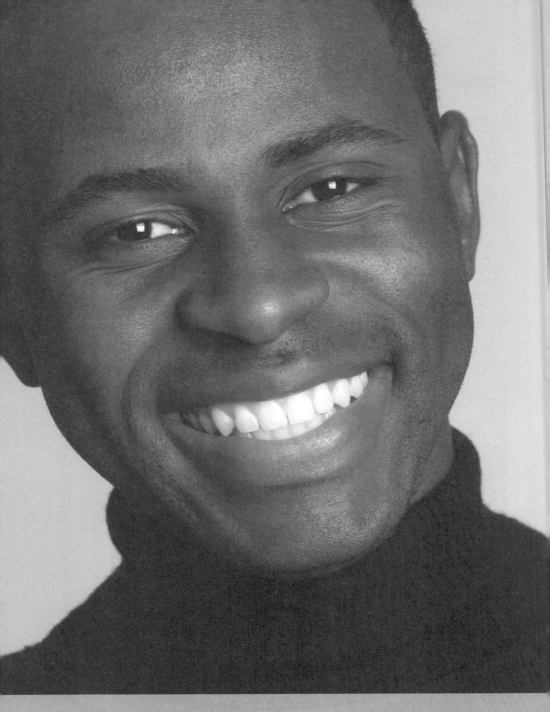

Chapter IV:
Creating a Beautiful Smile

Comprehensive Dental Rehabilitation

In designing and planning your full dental rehabilitation (major repair of teeth) many factors must be considered. These include current health of the teeth, health of the gums, and other systemic factors such as general health and habits. We also must consider esthetics (cosmetics), speech, chewing function, longevity, and personal desires. We must take into account facial esthetics, joint and muscle function, and durability and we must choose the proper dental materials to give you the look, function and durability you desire. Modern dentistry has many new and unique materials which may be incorporated into your final treatment plan, and proper use of these materials is essential for successful results.

Dentures and Partials

Dentures and partial dentures ("partials") are often the easiest and fastest way to restore smile, function and confidence. Especially if you have fought major dental problems and tooth loss over the 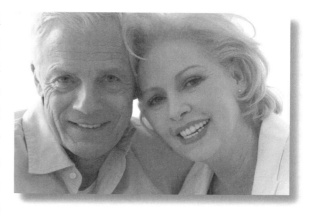 years, dentures and partials can be the easiest and most economical way for you to regain that smile, confidence and self image you desire. Our dentures are known for the change they have made in our patients' lives.

Please see our chapter on Dentures and Partial Dentures (p. 152) for more information.

Mini-Implants

Mini-Implants can be placed easily and comfortably in your jaws to act as artificial roots to support your dentistry. They can help make your dentures and partials so much more comfortable and functional. You will be amazed at how easily you can now wear dentures and partials, chew comfortably, and look great! For more information, please see our chapter on Implants (p. 112).

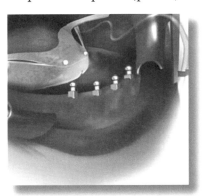
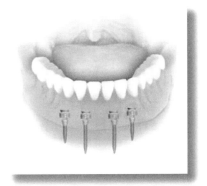

Ceramic Inlays & Porcelain Crowns

If all-porcelain fillings and crowns are your desire, here too, we can serve you. While porcelain crowns and partial crowns (inlays and onlays) are not right for all situations, especially for high-stress chewers, grinders, and clenchers, in many cases they are the most tooth-friendly, conservative dental restorations available. Using all-porcelain, we can often strengthen and save more of your tooth and precious enamel for years to come. All-porcelain crowns, where indicated, are beautiful and long-lasting. Please refer to our chapter on Crowns (p. 142) for more information.

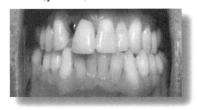
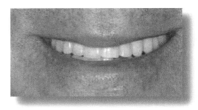

Implants, Crowns, & Bridges

Missing teeth detract from your smile, your chewing ability, and your dental health. Bridges to replace missing teeth have been our mainstay for many years; these consist of dental crowns on the supporting teeth (abutments) and a false tooth (pontic) to fill the missing tooth space(s). Cemented in place, a bridge replaces missing esthetics and function. In the last two decades, implants to replace missing teeth have been a wonder for those in need of tooth replacement. A titanium tooth-form cylinder is placed in the jawbone in a simple quick procedure. The implant fuses to the bone (osseointegrates) where it strengthens and stabilizes. It is then used as a support for an abutment (sub-structure) and crown, without involving unnecessary treatment on adjacent teeth. While more costly, implants are often the most ideal treatment to replace and restore teeth. They may also be used to support dentures and extensive full mouth rehabilitation (tooth replacement). Please see our chapters on Implants (p. 112), Crowns (p. 142), and Bridges (p. 148).

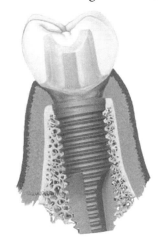

"I have been going to Dr. Finkel for over five years now, and he has been a great friend and doctor. I love his honesty and professionalism.

"All my visits have been very relaxing and fun. The staff is outstanding and very helpful.

"My teeth were in a terrible state and he has given me my smile back. Thank you, Dr. Finkel and staff for making my visits enjoyable."

Jennie

Periodontal (Gum) Plastic Surgery

A beautiful smile includes not just the teeth, but the lips and gums that frame your teeth. Too little gum (recession) or too much gum (a "gummy smile") can ruin the framing and the esthetics of your teeth and smile. If the gum has been lost around a tooth or teeth, we can graft back gum tissue to cover exposed roots, strengthen the gums, and decrease root sensitivity. If you show too much gum, we can reshape the gums with a simple surface procedure (gingivectomy) or, when necessary, an easy procedure to reshape the surface tissue and underlying supportive tissue. Our goal is your beautiful smile and strong, healthy gums for a great overall dental picture. Please see our chapter on Periodontal Disease and Treatment (p. 90).

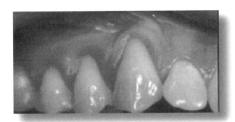 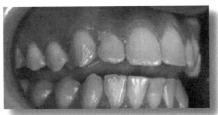

"After a few years away I found my way home to Dr. Finkel and his amazing staff. He is a wonderfully talented dentist who truly cares for his patients.

"After a procedure he calls after hours to check on your progress.

"Dr. Finkel has a gift and uses his talents to enhance others' lives through an exceptional dental practice. I will never stray again."

Amber

Materials Used for Tooth Restorations

The following information will help you select the type of tooth restorations you prefer to have placed, to restore the structure of individual teeth.

Your choices for fillings:

▪ **Good: Silver Amalgam**

Average longevity about 15 years, silver colored, low initial cost. Best used in small to medium sized restorations of posterior (back) teeth (premolars and molars). Resists redecay in deeper cavities and wears well, but does not strengthen teeth. Used in areas of difficult access and best for cavity (decay) -prone situations

▪ **Good: Composite Resin - direct** *(one-appointment placement)*

Average longevity 10-15 years, tooth colored, moderate cost. Best used in small to medium sized restorations for any teeth. Considered at this time to be competitive with silver amalgam. Esthetic, but may not resist redecay in deeper cavities. Can strengthen and help hold together a weakened tooth. As the composite resins continue to improve, they are becoming the filling material of choice; may not be as decay-resistant as amalgam. More difficult and time consuming to properly place; are therefore more costly (if done properly).

▪ **Better: Resin and ceramic lab-fabricated tooth-colored inlays and onlays**
(may be done as CAD-CAM (computer designed and manufactured) one- or two-appointment placement)

Average longevity (expected) 10- 15 years, tooth-colored, moderate to high initial cost. Best used in medium-sized restorations for posterior (back) teeth (premolars and molars). Can bond to and strengthen teeth. Durable and esthetic; wear very well, and should only be placed where proper bonding techniques are possible and where the tooth can be isolated from saliva and moisture during placement.

▪ Best: Gold Inlays and Onlays

Average longevity 20 years to life, gold colored, moderate to high initial cost. May be used in any sized restoration in any location where metal display is not objectionable. Not as esthetic, but the strongest, most durable of all tooth restorations. This is the best restoration for lifetime service and having a dental restoration last as long as possible. The intricacy and time of the dental treatment makes this the most costly filling technique. But the one that helps best save damaged teeth, giving longest term service and ultimately giving top value over your lifetime.

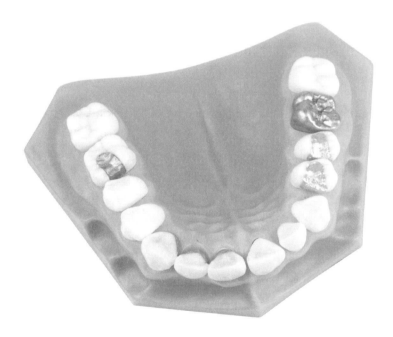

Where's the Wisdom in Removing Wisdom Teeth?

Believe it or not, our wisdom teeth don't give us much wisdom. In fact, they usually bring questions to mind.

We're often asked, "Why are wisdom teeth removed even if they don't hurt?"

Many times there are no symptoms of wisdom tooth trouble, but x-rays may show us that there is the potential for a serious problem or that other teeth in your mouth may be at risk for damage.

About 28% of wisdom teeth are impacted because the jaw is not big enough to accommodate them. These impacted wisdom teeth may grow sideways, break part way through the gum, or remain trapped beneath the gum and bone.

Bacteria and food can lodge under the flap of gum over the partially erupted tooth, causing infection in the gum. A cyst can form around the crown of the tooth and destroy the surrounding bone or neighboring teeth.

Because of their position, wisdom teeth are difficult to clean and are often victims of decay. The results of extensive orthodontic treatment can be ruined if your wisdom teeth crowd adjacent teeth, causing them to shift position.

If we spot a potential problem, we may recommend removing the wisdom tooth even before it is fully developed. It is easier to remove wisdom teeth at an early stage because the roots aren't fully formed or strongly planted in the jaw. That means that the sooner your wisdom teeth are removed, the easier the procedure and the smaller your risk of complications.

Please let us know right away if you have any obvious problems with your wisdom teeth. You can rely on our expertise to diagnose existing or potential problems caused by your wisdom teeth, whether you have symptoms or not.

Chapter V:
Orthodontics

Orthodontics: Why Straighten Teeth?

A beautiful smile is always associated with overall attractiveness, success, confidence, and happiness in life. Having a beautiful smile is one of the ways we show others that we have self-respect, self-confidence, and what it takes to get ahead. It has also been shown to aid in our attracting that perfect mate.

Surprisingly, a straight, even, smile is also highly associated with better health; straight teeth are easier to clean, have less gum infection, and are associated with heart health and lower rates of systemic disease. These associations are covered in the section on Periodontal Disease (p. 90) and in the section on The Oral-Systemic Connection (pp. 220-227).

Straight teeth also more properly and evenly support the bite for greater health of the teeth, jaw joints(TMJs), and biting muscles. A proper bite helps reduce the chances of "TMJ," headache and facial pain.

For these reasons, as well as improved ability to chew and speak, it is a good idea to orthodontically straighten crooked teeth and even-up the bite. Following is an overview of several techniques we use to accomplish this.

"I have remained a patient of Dr. Finkel, even after working for another dentist, because of his quality of work and commitment to excellence."

Joanne

Power-Prox 6 Month Orthodontics

The PowerProx 6 Month Braces system of orthodontics is designed for those who want rapid improvement of their smile (front teeth) without changing the over-all bite or jaw position relationship. In about six months, we can often align and level the front teeth for a more attractive smile without invasive and expensive dental procedures.

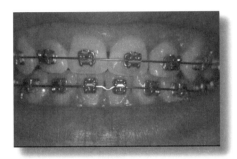 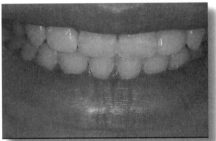

Invisalign Braces

Invisalign is a relatively new approach to orthodontics (braces). Invisalign is an orthodontic technique which replaces the wires and brackets of traditional braces with clear, nearly-invisable, aligner trays so no-one else ever needs to know you are having your teeth straightened. The clear trays are removable, comfortable, and esthetic; even during social situations, they can be worn with confidence.

What is Invisalign?

For many years, dentistry has used clear retainers, "essix" retainers and many forms of clear trays to correct minor tooth alignment problems. They have been used to close spaces between teeth, straighten crowded teeth, and correct crooked teeth, but they were mainly used for minor tooth movement, minor corrections, and smaller segments of the dental arch.

Invisalign has expanded the use of these clear aligner trays to include more significant tooth movement and full-arch orthodontic correction. You can confidently smile during and after your

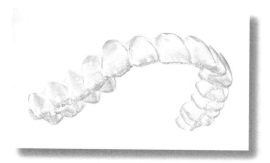

treatment; the clear trays are nearly invisible (Invisalign = "Invisible Aligners", get it?) The series of clear aligner trays gradually moves your teeth to your final desired result and usual treatment time is about a year, with dentist visits every 4-6 weeks. Each tray moves the teeth a small amount; the result is a series of corrections adding up to the final result. Eating, brushing, and flossing can continue as normal.

What are the benefits of Invisalign?

Invisalign is used to correct tooth spacing in wider arches, tooth crowding in narrow arches, tooth rotations, and many other orthodontic problems previously only treatable with traditional bands, braces and wires. The benefits include healthier gums (straighter teeth are easier to clean) and easier home care (flossing and brushing are less trouble).

Tooth wear is often decreased; mis-aligned teeth have abnormal wear because the teeth take pressure unevenly. Out-of-line teeth hit harder, break, and wear more rapidly; once aligned, that abnormal wear is decreased. Also, aligned teeth that function well together often result in less clenching and grinding (bruxing) and less tooth wear.

When should we not use Invisalign?

Invisalign orthodontics is not for every patient; fixed orthodontics (brackets and wires) allows the dentist to "grab hold" of the teeth and move tooth crowns and roots into the most stable alignment. Brackets and wires may be more effective for subtle tooth position corrections requiring more complex forces and movements. Certain more complex orthodontic situations require the control afforded by fixed brackets and wires, and some corrections can be handled more quickly with fixed orthodontics.

Orthodontic problems often best treated with traditional braces include jaw-joint problems, facial growth and development problems, and problems involving one arch of teeth (upper or lower) being totally out of fit with the other. Orthodontic problems where the dental arches are incorrectly placed in the face or where there are major discrepancies between teeth, dental arches, and the face are usually outside the scope of Invisalign treatment.

Invisalign treatment is usually easiest and best for those orthodontic situations in which no major facial corrections are required, the upper and lower dental arches fit fairly well together, the jaw joints work well, and there are no major tooth spacing/crowding discrepancies.

How does Invisalign work?

The original Invisalign lacked some control of the teeth during treatment. The latest version of Invisalign offers greater ability to "grab hold" of the tooth crowns and roots. This control results in greater treatment accuracy, greater treatment speed, and greater treatment stability.

We start treatment with patient photographs, x-rays, and impressions. This information is then coordinated with desired treatment results, and the impressions are computer-scanned to form a virtual (computer) model of the beginning tooth positions. Sophisticated computer models and algorithms project a series of coordinated small tooth movements that, added together, give the final orthodontic results desired. Virtual dental models are created for each step of treatment, and computer-generated aligner trays, using SLA (Stereo Lithography) are made for each step with the final goal in mind.

How do you wear Invisalign Aligners?

These progressive aligner trays are worn for about two weeks each, until the teeth are moved into a position ready for the next tray. Sometimes the first step, prior to the first tray, is bonding onto certain teeth a small series of tooth-colored "buttons" for greater control: These attachments allow the trays to exert greater control and more exact forces to achieve the desired result. The attachments are then removed after treatment.

Each aligned tray must be worn for the full prescribed time each day and for the full period of days or weeks each is indicated. Failure to wear the trays for the proper time each day and the full number of days will slow treatment and compromise your results. Lack of patient compliance will doom your Invisalign treatment to failure. If your next aligner tray does not fit well to place (teeth not moving well or trays not worn enough), you may need to use the prior aligner tray for more time.

Once the full series of aligner trays is completed, more trays may be necessary for refinement of results. Sometimes mid-course corrections may be indicated, using a fresh series of aligner trays. At the end of treatment, attachments will be removed, and retainers will be designed and fabricated. Retainers, though strong, do wear and break (and are lost) over time, and will require a small fee to remake. Failure to wear retainers or have bonded retention (retainer) wires will result in relapse of a successful Invisalign result back toward your original orthodontic condition.

Properly diagnosed, planned, and executed, Invisalign can truly help you achieve that smile you have always wanted!

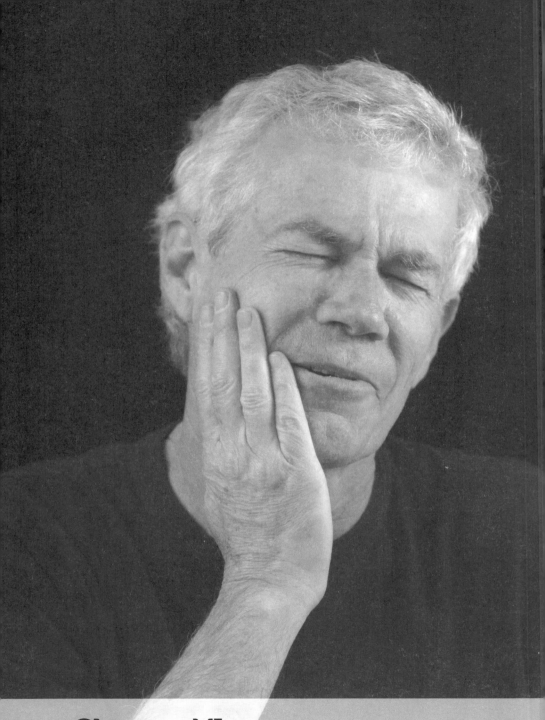

Chapter VI:
TMJ, Headache and Facial Pain

Bruxism, Clenching, and Grinding

What is Bruxism? What is Clenching and Grinding?

Some people bite their fingernails. Others spend hours at the gym. There are many ways, deliberate or unconscious, adaptive or unhealthy, of responding to and coping with stress. If your way involves habitually clenching or grinding your teeth, you are engaging in bruxism.

Bruxism is the habit of clenching and grinding the teeth. Clenching means you tightly hold your top and bottom teeth together. Grinding occurs when you slide your teeth back and forth over each other.

People who suffer from bruxism may experience the following:

- Headaches
- Sore Jaw
- Wear and breaking of teeth
- Frequent toothaches
- Facial pain
- Worn or fractured tooth enamel
- Earache and Vertigo (loss of balance)
- Insomnia (inability to go to sleep or to stay asleep)

Why is Bruxism bad?

What's wrong with a little tooth gnashing, you might ask? For one, enough bruxism can damage the teeth. It can also tire jaw muscles and cause them to go into spasm. The spasm causes pain, which in turn causes more spasm. The end result of this spasm-pain-spasm cycle may eventually be a temporomandibular (TM) disorder, a problem with the way the jaw muscles, ligaments, bones, and joints work together.

The tendency to "brux" can be other than stress-related. Malocclusion, a problem with the way teeth fit together when the mouth is closed, can also trigger persistent tooth clenching, and ultimately result in a TM disorder ("TMJ" or "TMD").

How Does Bruxism Damage Teeth?

When we clench and grind our teeth, daily and nightly, the grinding action of the opposing teeth against each other causes the tooth enamel to wear, chip, and fracture. As the enamel parts of the tooth wear away, they become thinner and thinner, weaker and weaker. Enamel may then chip off in pieces, so the ongoing wear and chipping cause the teeth to become pointed, sharp, broken, and shorter. Front teeth may become thinner, with sharp, jagged edges, and back teeth may become flatter. Teeth are formed with rounded contours; any sharp, flat, jagged edges are the result of wear and breakage.

Grinding and clenching can also crack and split teeth; the forces of the muscles contracting can put so much pressure on the teeth that whole pieces are broken off, especially if the tooth is already weakened by previous cavities and the resultant fillings. If the forces are too great and too vertical, then the tooth may split vertically in the body and roots of the tooth.

What is Cracked Tooth Syndrome?

If the split in the tooth is still shallow, then the tooth can be saved with a crown. If the split goes deeper into the pulp (nerve) of the tooth, then the tooth may be salvageable with a root canal, core, and crown. If the split has entered the body and roots of the tooth, then the split will form a line that oral bacteria can always travel along into the gum and bone. This tooth will be lost; no amount of dental treatment can save it for the long-term.

Cracked (split) teeth can often be difficult to diagnose and may present puzzling and intermittent symptoms that can confound the dentist and patient. Diagnosis requires special tests and elimination of other diagnoses.

What is the Treatment for Cracked Tooth Syndrome?

Cracked teeth also create a dilemma in treatment. To determine if the tooth is salvageable, treatment (often including root canal) must be begun to determine if the crack is shallow enough for treatment to succeed or deep enough that extraction becomes the proper choice. It is possible that even proper treatment can appear to give a good prognosis, only to still have the tooth fail and require extraction at a later date. Each case of split (cracked) tooth syndrome will present its own challenges, and successful treatment may be a matter of relative odds based on initial findings, not guaranteed long-term success.

What are Abfractions and Abfractive Lesions?

When we clench and grind, daily and nightly, we also cause the teeth to bend and flex at their narrowest part; the neck of the tooth where the crown meets the root. As the tooth flexes, the crystals of tooth structure are weakened at this area right at the gum in a process known as abfraction. Engineers know this as stress corrosion. In abfraction, these weakened crystals at the tooth neck are then abraded (brushed) away by toothbrush and toothpaste. Hard, vigorous, horizontal toothbrushing increases this loss of tooth structure, and the addition of abrasive toothpaste increases this loss of tooth structure by seven to ten times. Consumption of acid drinks like sodas, sports drinks, energy

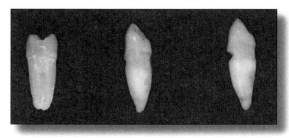

drinks, and acidic juices further weakens and erodes these crystals of tooth structure, accelerating the tooth loss.

All such abfractive lesions at the neck of the tooth have some component of tooth flexure (stress corrosion), toothbrush/toothpaste abrasion, and acid attack. It is often difficult to decide what percentage each contributes to the damage.

Proper treatment involves restoration of the abfractive lesions with fillings or crowns to protect and stiffen the tooth, and correction of the etiology (cause).

This may involve:

- Change in toothbrushing technique
- Change in or elimination of toothpaste
- Elimination of acidic drinks and foods
- Use of fluorides to strengthen the tooth structure against acid attack
- Bite adjustments to minimize grinding stresses on individual teeth
- Nightguard use to minimize stress/and tooth flexure at nights
- Dayguard use to protect from daily grinding
- Biofeedback to minimize grinding damage
- Simple tooth restoration involving bonded fillings to protect and stiffen teeth, possibly requiring periodic replacement when tooth flexure causes de-bonding
- More involved crowns (with cores) to restore strength and structure to the involved teeth

Bruxism can cause severe tooth damage and tooth loss. It can also contribute in multiple ways to damage from other causes and should be recognized and treated.

How do you develop Bruxism?

Bruxism can develop at any age, and children, as well as adults, can have the habit of grinding their teeth. Stressful situations, sleep disorders, abnormal bite, and crooked or missing teeth may be responsible. Childhood airway problems from allergies and tonsil/adenoid involvement can cause mouth-breathing which changes tongue and cheek muscle activity and results in narrowed dental arches and teeth which do not fit correctly together. Continued airway problems and occlusal (bite) disharmony increases unwanted dental grinding.

We can diagnose bruxism by looking for unusual wear spots on your teeth, and regular dental checkups are important to detect damage in the early stages. We can treat wear on teeth and facial pain that may result from bruxism. Bruxism may be an indicator of obstructive sleep apnea and the body's attempt to open a closed-down airway by increasing tongue and jaw-muscle activity. Many anti-psychotic and anti-depressant drugs can cause extreme clenching and grinding, leading to TMJ problems.

How is Bruxism treated?

Stress reduction, nutritional factors, and exercises may help. Nightguards are helpful for bruxism caused by sleep disorders, crooked or missing teeth, or stress. Custom-made to fit your teeth, the night-guard slips over the upper or lower teeth and prevents contact between them. It helps relieve some of the pressure of grinding or clenching, which can damage jaw joints, muscles, and teeth. Some nightguards are designed to spread the bite forces over many teeth and unload the TM joints; these usually fit over all of the upper or all of the lower teeth. In certain situations, the nightguard may have two parts; one covering the upper teeth and one covering the lowers.

Some nightguards may separate the back teeth; the biting muscles cannot fully activate when the back teeth are apart. When biting only on the front teeth, the human bite system inhibits contraction of the biting muscles. The goal of these appliances is to inhibit activation of the bite muscles, unload the jaw joint(s), and have any residual grinding occur on the plastic of the guard, not on the teeth (now protected). Depending upon when the bulk of the bruxing occurs, these appliances can be designed to be worn during sleep or at various times during the day.

Stress-induced grinding can often be dealt with by reducing or eliminating the stress itself. Counseling can be used along with other forms of treatment for bruxism. Bio-feedback, a relaxation technique that teaches you to control the tension in various parts of your body with the aid of an electronic monitoring machine, can help reduce jaw muscle tension and the urge to grind as well. If bruxism arises from malocclusion (bad bite), the problem can be treated with orthodontics (braces) and other dental procedures such as occlusal (bite) adjustment of your teeth. See the section on Full Mouth Occlusal (Bite) Adjustment (p. 84).

During your initial examination in our office, we evaluate for grinding or clenching habits, and for clicking noises as your jaw opens and closes. Additionally, we observe and note excessive wear of individual teeth in your mouth. As always, we welcome any questions you have concerning bruxism and your particular bite.

> *"Dr. Finkel has been a great dentist. I love my smile, and he and his friendly staff make me feel like family.*
>
> *"I highly recommend Dr. Finkel to my family and friends!"*
>
> *Sonja*

Head, Neck & Face Pain – TM Disorders: TMJ & TMD

Most of us can chew, yawn, open, and close our mouths effortlessly; our jaws and surrounding facial muscles work together in harmony. Any disruption in this intricate, harmonious relationship between muscles and bones, however, can trigger the chronic facial discomfort of a temporomandibular (TM) disorder. These disorders are often characterized by a vicious cycle of muscle spasm, pain, tenderness, tissue damage, more muscle spasm, and further injury. They are known as "TMJ" or "TMD" Problems, "TMJ" or "TMD".

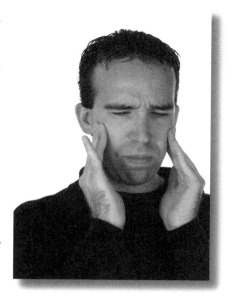

What is the TMJ and what is "TMJ"?

The temporomandibular joint (TMJ) is the joint that connects the jaw to the skull. For a long time, dentists thought all TM disorders were caused solely by malocclusions or problems with the way the teeth fit together, causing pain and dysfunction in the TMJ (joint) and surrounding muscles. We now know that TM disorders are really a group of several different disorders, each with unique causes and each requiring unique treatments, but all related to how the jaws, joints, muscles, and teeth work together. "TMJ" or "TMD" are terms used as shorthand for this group of painful disorders which are by no means rare. An estimated 20+ million Americans suffer from them and each patient with "TMJ" needs to know that his or her pain has a specific diagnosis. "TMJ" is not a diagnosis. If you saw an orthopedist for a painful leg joint, you would be disappointed to be told you have "knee", or with a painful upper limb, to be told you have "arm."

Similarly, a diagnosis of "TMJ" is a non-specific description of pain in this area. To begin solving and treating your pain and dysfunction problem requires evaluation and diagnosis of specific ailment(s) of the joints, muscles, nerves, ligaments, tendons, teeth, habits and function, prior to targeted treatment and therapy.

What are the signs and symptoms of TMJ/TMD Disorders?

Because of the broad spectrum of symptoms associated with TMJ Disorder, it is often referred to as the "great imposter." While there are many symptoms of TMJ Disorder, many patients do not associate their discomfort and pain with TMJ Disorder and are often left undiagnosed. Referred pain from the temporomandibular joint and muscles can mimic ear or sinus infections, and cause pain in the head, neck, shoulders, back, or eyes. Some of the most common symptoms are the following:

- Pain in or around the ear, often spreading to the face
- Tenderness of the jaw muscles
- Clicking or popping noise when one opens or closes the mouth
- Difficulty in opening one's mouth
- Jaws that "get stuck," "lock," or "go out"
- Pain brought on by yawning, chewing, or opening the mouth widely
- Headaches or neck aches; especially disabling pain in the neck and base of the skull

- Ringing or stuffiness in the ears, or inner ear problems

- Dizziness, vertigo, or balance problems

- Increased nervousness

- Gross fatigue, aggravated by pain-induced sleep disorders

- Dementia; which appears to be aggravated by a bad bite and resultant improper brain function

How do we diagnose the specific cause of TMJ?

We can determine the cause of your symptoms by conducting a series of diagnostic tests. These may include a complete medical history, clinical examination, X-rays, and casts (models) of your teeth. We may refer you to a physician or other specialist. To help with the diagnosis of your problem, we may involve a neurologist, ENT physician, rheumatologist, chiropractor, physical therapist, and massage therapist. This procedure may seem time-consuming, but proper diagnosis is an important step prior to treatment. It can save time and money by ensuring that you receive the treatment appropriate for your particular problem.

Most of the diagnosis of TMJ comes from patient history and direct one-on-one physical examination. Many of our questions may seem picky and unrelated, and much of what we ask may seem boring. A thorough patient history gives us about 50% of our diagnostic information, and most of the rest of our needed information comes from the physical examination of the joints, muscles, ligaments, tendons, nerves, teeth, and surrounding structures. We also check jaw movement, joint function, muscle activity, range of jaw motion, location of pain, type of pain, and pain-aggravating factors. Radiographs (x-rays) of the jaws, M.R.I.s, C.A.T. scans, and other medical imaging give us additional information as needed.

We evaluate diet, lifestyle, work-habits, personal habits, and life stressors for "activating" factors and "perpetuating" factors which initiate and continue the pain. We diagnose and analyze within the "bucket theory" of pain and dysfunction. That is, we are all designed to function within a range of physical, physiological, emotional, nutritional, and functional limits (the "walls" of our "bucket"). When our bucket is filled to capacity with these stressors and begins to "overflow," that overflow represents the pain and dysfunction of exceeding our individual design parameters. We search for those physical, mental, and functional stressors which exceed our ability to "cope" and which result in exactly the pain and symptoms (the "overflow") of this disorder.

To help you regain health, we can then "raise the walls" of the bucket by helping you improve your nutrition, physical habits, coping skills, and health so you (and your "bucket") have higher walls, greater capacity, and greater ability to handle life without overflowing into symptoms.

We also seek to find and limit those factors and stressors flowing into (filling) the bucket, by helping you change or avoid work habits, personal habits, emotional habits, food habits, and physical habits that threaten to continually raise the stressor level inside (fill) your bucket to overflowing. Simultaneously, we work to raise your ability to cope and physically handle "stuff" ("raising the bucket walls") and to lower the stressors (inflow), so we eliminate pain and dysfunction (no "overflow").

What are the causes of TMJ Disorders?

Causes of TMJ problems include history of facial trauma and/or motor vehicle accidents, sleep disorders with clenching and grinding, obstructive sleep apnea, medication side-effects, medical disorders (listed below), and neural (nerve) disorders. Heart disease, sinus infection, spinal problems, improper nutrition, inadequate hydration (fluids), and stress are also contributing factors. Harmful habits are a major cause of TMJ pain and include bruxing, pipe-smoking, pencil-biting, and gum-chewing.

Gum chewing in females, especially young women, has been shown to cause TM joint popping, clicking, and pain. The repeated chewing trauma causes internal derangement of the joint; the inner parts of the joint do not work together in harmony. In many women, continued gum chewing results in permanent joint damage, improper function, and future TMJ problems. Gum-chewing is harmful to the joints and should be avoided.

Oral habits such as clenching the teeth or grinding the teeth (bruxism) can cause TMJ pain. These habits can tire the muscles and cause them to go into spasm. The spasm causes pain which, in turn, causes more spasm. The end result of this spasm-pain-spasm cycle may eventually be a TMJ Disorder.

Problems in the way the teeth fit together, or bite, can initiate TMJ Disorders. Improperly aligned teeth can sometimes place the chewing muscles under stress and cause them to go into spasm, thus setting off the harmful cycle described earlier.

Frequently, oral habits and bite problems work together to cause TMJ Disorders.

Example 1:

Paula is under a great deal of pressure from work. She develops a habit of grinding her teeth while sleeping. This causes muscle spasm and, eventually, pain and tenderness in her jaw muscles. Because of these problems, a slight change in the position of Paula's jaw occurs, and her teeth no longer fit together correctly. She develops a new chewing pattern, and this increases the muscle spasm.

Example 2:

Ever since he was a boy, David, has had teeth that do not fit together correctly when his mouth is closed. This never seemed to be much of a problem for him, but now his bad bite triggers tooth clenching and causes his chewing muscles to function incorrectly. Muscle spasm occurs, and pain limits the normal range of David's jaw movements. As a result, David's chewing pattern changes, and this contributes to his TMJ symptoms.

How do airway problems cause TMJ problems?

TMJ problems are often caused by occlusal (bite) disharmony which was caused by childhood airway problems. Many kids have nasal congestion due to allergies. They may be allergic to pollens, environmental allergens, dairy, chocolate, corn, wheat, nuts, sodas, etc. Allergies cause nasal congestion and enlargement of the tonsils and adenoids, as well as difficulty in breathing through the nose resulting in mouth-breathing. Infections of the tonsils and adenoids cause further enlargement, more nasal blockage, and increased mouth-breathing. Mouth-breathing moves the tongue into an abnormal position, which does not support proper dental arch development and activates the cheek muscles to constrict the width of the dental arches which now cannot develop into their normal form.

The jaw must move backward to bite properly, and the tongue must move forward to breath properly. The patient now has teeth that do not fit properly together and becomes a chronic mouth-breather. So, early airway problems cause bite problems which then cause TMJ problems. These same patients then also have airway problems which cause Obstructive Sleep Apnea, a deadly affliction. Early treatment of allergies and airway problems can help avoid TMJ dysfunction and sleep apnea.

What are other dental causes of TMJ Disorders?

TMJ Disorders can be initiated (begun) by a single tooth, filling, or crown which is too high for the normal bite or an abscessed tooth causing pain on biting. TMJ can also be initiated by dental arches (teeth) that do not properly support the joints and muscles. The upper and lower arches of teeth may be misaligned so that closing the teeth together causes torquing (twisting) or over-closing of the TM (jaw) joints, and spasm of the face and jaw muscles to compensate. Dentures can lack proper bite support for the jaws, so the airway is closed down; and bruxism occurs as the body attempts to activate the airway-opening muscles. Therefore, improper bite of all the teeth, or of a single tooth, can cause joint and muscle issues and can initiate TMJ problems, and an abscessed tooth can initiate or duplicate these problems. Many anti-psychotic and anti-depressant drugs can cause extreme clenching and grinding, leading to TMJ problems.

What are some other medical issues which show up as "TMJ"?

Other medical issues which present as TMJ-type pain are:

- Sinus infection or throat infection
- Ear infection or inner-ear disturbance
- Fibromyalgia or chronic fatigue syndrome
- Sleep disorder or obstructive sleep apnea
- Nocturnal Bruxism (nightly clenching and grinding)
- Neurological disorders or medication-induced muscle problems
- Rheumatoid arthritis or osteoarthritis
- Cancer or cancer-related diseases
- Metabolic disorders or auto-immune diseases

Treatment for TMJ Disorders

Dentists use a wide range of treatments to manage TMJ Disorders, from drug therapy with muscle relaxants to surgery. Other components of treatment programs for TMJ Disorders include soft-food diets, massage, moist heat applications, bite adjustments, bite appliances, physical therapy, and relaxation exercises.

Some common methods of treating TMJ Disorders are:

Elimination of spasm and pain: This can be done by applying moist heat to the face with exercises, using prescribed muscle relaxants or other medications, massaging the muscles, and eating soft, non-chewy foods. Bite plates or occlusal (bite) splints may be required to relax the muscles, to decompress the jaw joints, and to protect the teeth. This appliance, known as a "M.O.R.A.", is a Mandibular Orthopedic Repositioning Appliance and may be used full-time daily, nightly, or in some combination to help the muscles relax.

Counseling or biofeedback/relaxation training: Many times, counseling is used along with other forms of treatment. If emotional stress is the factor that causes clenching or grinding of the teeth, that stress should be reduced or eliminated. Biofeedback can also be helpful in reducing muscle tension in the neck, jaws, and face. Physical therapy, nutritional supplementation, life-style guidance, and coping skills may help.

Changes in lifestyle and harmful habits: TMJ therapy may include improvements in nutrition, fluid intake, sleep hygiene, and daily exercise; special jaw and neck exercises may also be prescribed for your condition. It is important to avoid stressful neck positions at work and home. Posture training and breathing training may be needed, as may avoiding harmful habits such as overly-aggressive chewing, hard foods, and gum-chewing. Gum chewing should always be avoided to minimize trauma to the TM joints and stress on the muscles.

Correcting the way the teeth fit together: If your bite is incorrect or uneven, it can be adjusted by selective bite adjustment of the teeth. Orthodontic appliance (braces) and other dental procedures may also be used to reduce problems caused by incorrect tooth contact (improperly aligned teeth). Correction of the problem can involve treating the bite of one or of several teeth. Correction can also involve braces or surgery to move all the teeth into a bite position that properly supports the joints and muscles of the face.

Bite appliances: A MORA, or bite splint, may be used to help diagnose a bite problem, aid in healing of the joints and muscles, and provide long-term support of the joints and muscles in the correct position. The MORA may be initially worn full-time, out only to eat and clean, for diagnosis and to aid in initial healing. After initial (Phase I) therapy, it may be worn nightly and full-time during periods of stress.

All or some of the above treatments will likely be employed in combination for both short-term healing and long-term maintenance of health. Both short-term and long-term treatment will also likely involve support of other health professionals and "adjunctive" lifestyle changes.

What about long-term treatment?

The above-noted treatments are part of Phase I therapy to diagnose problems, decrease pain, and restore function. During this phase, diagnosis and treatment are like peeling an onion; as one level (layer) of therapy is diagnosed and treated, the next layer becomes available to be addressed. Once the issues of pain and dysfunction are resolved, often involving consultation with other medical professionals, and the patient is able to function more normally, then the issue of long-term therapy is addressed. Phase II therapy is employed to maintain this regained level of health and comfort and may be as simple as nightly wear of your appliance with life-style changes or as complex as rebuilding your bite with orthodontics (braces) and complex restorative dentistry. Please see Phase I TMJ Therapy and Phase II TMJ Therapy sections below.

Surgery: If muscle spasm has occurred for long periods, the TM joint itself may become injured or arthritic. In addition, the hard and soft tissues of the TMJ may slip out of normal position because of trauma, such as a blow to the head, motor vehicle accident, or other injury. Occasionally, in severe cases such as these, surgery may be needed to correct the TMJ problem as part of long-term, Phase II, therapy.

Generally, our goal is to reduce the stress on the teeth, muscles, and joints to allow healing and pain relief. We then, with nutrition and lifestyle modifications, try to give the body greater capacity to deal with negative stressors so it can better resist those things which otherwise cause pain. This way, we increase the *height of the walls* of your *bucket*.

In summary, our goal is to relieve the pain and dysfunction of your TMJ Disorder and allow you to heal. We will use special exercises, nutritional support, dental appliances, physical therapy, lifestyle changes, and medications as indicated. We may involve chiropractors, physical therapists, physical-medicine specialists, and massage therapists as part of our team. We then need to provide you with options for long-term, Phase II, therapy to help maintain any needed changes in jaw support and bite position.

Why is the TMJ evaluation so detailed?

Temporomandibular joint dysfunction and myofascial (muscle-tissue) pain can mimic other dental and medical problems. The diagnosis is very important because some of the medical problems that have similar headache or neck-ache symptoms can be life threatening; for example, intracranial tumor or coronary heart disease. You can help by giving the doctor a detailed medical and family history including a history of any food or drug allergies. Treatment for TM Joint/Myofascial disorders can be lengthy and frustrating. You should inform your doctor about changes in jaw function; the best therapeutic improvement is a result of good patient-doctor communication. Please call our office anytime there is a problem or question about treatment.

How long should TMJ Therapy take?

Treatment time can vary widely. In general, the treatment plan will be more lengthy and complicated if the symptoms are severe or if the problem has existed for a long time. Mild clicking with occasional muscle spasm headache may be successfully treated within a few weeks or months, but a long-standing arthritic joint disorder may require surgery, dental prosthetics, orthodontics, and/or extensive restorative treatment procedures.

What is Phase I TMJ Therapy?

Phase I (Splint, Orthotic, or MORA) Therapy is a diagnostic procedure attempting to establish proper function of the jaws, muscles, and joints, and to determine the jaw position which maintains normal function. During Phase I, we attempt to make the joints and muscles comfortable and pain free; multiple visits and adjustments are required as joint/ muscles inflammation decreases and muscle spasm subsides. Procedures may involve bite adjustments (see section on Occlusal Adjustment [p. 84]), TENS (muscle-pulsing) therapy, trigger point (muscle) injections, etc; at separate fees. Duration and cost of Phase I therapy with your dentist is usually 6-18 months and in the range of $3000 to $7000 (in 2012).

What is Phase II TMJ Therapy?

Phase II Therapy is projected to stabilize and hold the jaws at the position determined by Phase I; cost and specific procedures can be determined only if and when Phase I has been completed and the needs of your jaw position and bite support evaluated. Phase II therapies are separate procedures with separate fees from Phase I treatments and may include any of the following:

a. No further treatment (i.e. no Phase II Therapy needed)

b. Night time wear only of the appliance

c. Dietary and habit modification

d. Bite (occlusal) adjustments

e. Crowns and bridges to establish the bite and/or replace missing teeth

f. Dentures/partial dentures to establish the bite and replace missing teeth

g. Orthodontics (braces)

h. A long term (overlay) appliance on the teeth

i. Surgical correction (in certain limited cases)

Phase II fees can be established at the completion of Phase I Therapy.

What are the possible complications of TMJ Therapy?

We will make our best effort to diagnose and treat any TMJ Disorder with timely and cost-effective methods. The most proven and conservative techniques will be used. However, you should be aware that there is much debate in the scientific literature on the most effective techniques and/or combination of treatment modalities. These include, but are not limited to, prosthetic splints, restorative and prosthetic dental procedures, surgical dental procedures, TM Joint surgery, biofeedback, phonophoresis, iontophoresis, transcutaneous electrical nerve stimulation (TENS), minimal electroneural stimulation (MENS), acupuncture, muscle trigger-point injections, hypnosis, psychological counseling, orthodontic and orthopedic appliances. Orthodontic, orthopedic, and prosthetic appliances may, theoretically, be swallowed or inhaled, though this is highly unlikely with the appliances we now use. Our modern appliances are designed for safe, effective, long-term use.

Are there other precautions I should be aware of?

Some TMJ symptoms may temporarily become worse with treatment. Patients with long-standing arthritic joint disease or traumatic injury can demonstrate more severe symptoms during the initial stages of therapy.

As with any form of medical or dental treatment, unusual complications can and do occur. Broken or loosened teeth, dislodged dental restorations, mouth sores, periodontal problems, root resorption, non-vital (needing root canal) teeth, muscle spasms, ear and back problems, and numbness are all possible occurrences.

As with any medical treatments, guarantees of success can not be given; often this problem can be successfully managed but not cured. Failure to follow recommended treatment will certainly hamper the results and decrease the possibility of a successful therapeutic outcome.

Evaluation and treatment of TMJ disorders is certainly one of the most complex disciplines of dentistry. Experience, education, dedication and perseverance on our part can certainly help us improve your comfort and quality of life.

Neuromuscular Dentistry & Power Bite Splints

Dr. Finkel studied with Dr. Barnie Jankelson and Dr. Janet Travell, two of the doctors/researchers whose work formed the basis of Neuromuscular Dentistry, Myofascial Pain Therapy and "TMJ" treatment. Dr. Finkel can determine what type of TMJ/headache pain therapy is right for you and when your dentistry should be performed in Centric, Bio-Centric, Neuromuscular, or accommodated bite position.

We can also develop for you a neuromuscular "power" splint to help increase your athletic performance.

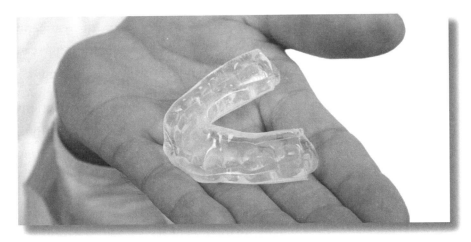

"Before I came to see Dr. Finkel, I was very self-conscious about my smile, which in turn made me feel bad about myself. Now, after many visits and wonderful people, and a very special Dr. Magic Man, I can talk and smile with ease.

"Thanks for giving me a big part of my life back."

Nancy

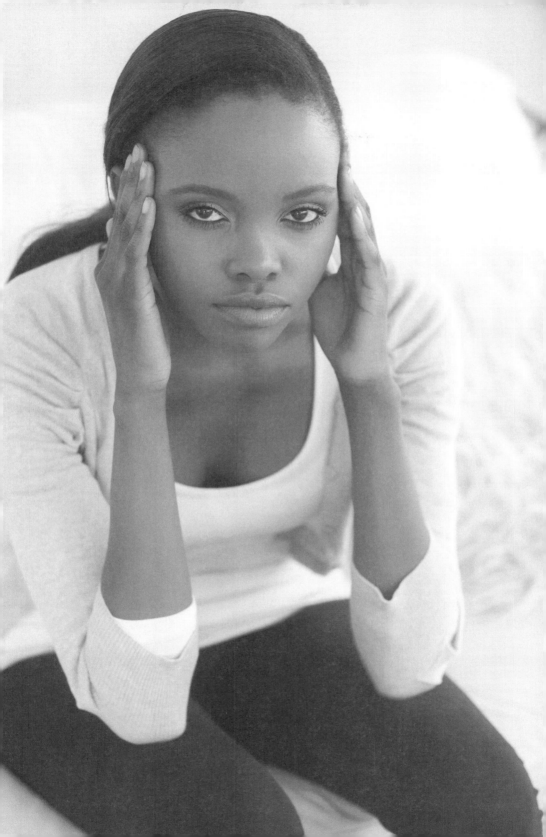

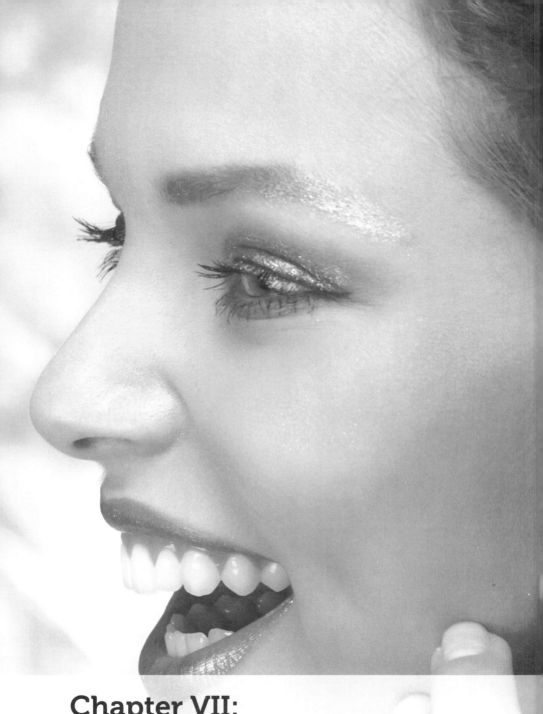

Chapter VII:
Full Mouth Occlusal
(Bite) Adjustment

Full-Mouth Occusal (Bite) Adjustment

The "perfect" bite for humans occurs when the jaw hinges (condyles) are evenly centered in both the right and left jaw joints (Temporomandibular joints or TM Joints) and, in this most natural position, the teeth come together evenly with no premature contacts (prematurities or deflective contacts) which cause the jaw to move or the jaw muscles to activate unevenly. Each human being has a slightly different centered (centric) jaw position, but one which is native, or natural to that individual.

What is centric jaw position?

The centric jaw position may be established by several different means, according to which school of thought the dentist follows. The goal of each school of thought is for the jaw to find its natural centric TM Joint position which is one of maximum comfort, function, and stability for that individual. In this ideal centric jaw position, several things occur:

1. The jaw joints are in their most natural, stable position.

2. This jaw position is repeatable and standard for that person.

3. In this position, when the jaw closes, all teeth hit evenly with no uneven forces on any teeth.

4. In this position, all teeth hit evenly with forces in line with the teeth, so they take biting forces at the correct angle.

5. In this centric jaw position, all teeth hit evenly, so the jaw is not deflected or moved to get all teeth to touch, and all teeth touch without the jaw joints being moved out of their centric positions.

6. All biting muscles activate evenly, with proper electrical (nerve) activity. No biting muscles contract before or with greater force than its mirror twin muscle on the other side of the face.

Why centric?

Unless all of these six conditions occur, there is one or more teeth contacting before the others so that the jaw must deviate or deflect from its centered position to get all the teeth to contact (bite). This deflective first tooth contact causes the jaw to move into an "eccentric" position, straining the joints, muscles, and teeth. The body and brain quickly learn to "dislike" these first erroneous contacts and to adopt an "avoidance bite" to bypass them. This bite, though wrong, feels to us like the natural bite; it is the only bite we know.

Because the bite is incorrect, unconscious clenching, grinding, and straining can damage the teeth, joints, and muscles. The shifted bite can cause: grinding forces which break teeth, excess pressure on front teeth, headaches, facial pain, and TM Joint problems. As long as there is no evidence of tooth grinding, excessive tooth wear, dental damage, headaches, facial pain, or joint problems we usually leave the bite as is, with no correction or change.

If, however, any of these problems are evident, the bite should be corrected with bite adjustment (occlusal equilibration), orthodontics (braces), or dental restoration to even up the bite and properly support the teeth, muscles and joints. Also, if any significant dental treatment is to be done, you do not want your dentistry to perpetuate and "lock-in" a bad bite. Even if no trouble now, it may cause problems later, after you have spent much money on your dentistry and you are kept in this bad bite.

Also, very importantly, we need to know the starting base position of your teeth and jaw from which to design the bite of your restorations (fillings and crowns) and back to where we adjust as your dentistry is being completed. Without this accurate base position to work from and back to, we can lose our direction in your dentistry and not know where to adjust to for your comfort, stability, and dental health.

To restore someone's teeth without a "home base" is like building a house on a shifting foundation or building a highway bridge where all its supports are on shifting sands. Successful dental treatment requires a stable foundation!

How do we find our dental "Home Base" for treatment?

To achieve these goals of centric jaw position coincident with even tooth contact and balanced forces within the teeth, muscle and joints, we often perform a bite adjustment or "occlusal equilibration." To accomplish this goal, we may first settle the joints and relax the muscles with an "anterior jig" (an anterior bite jig or deprogrammer) for some time prior to our adjusting (equilibrating) the bite. We may have the patient wear a special anterior deprogramming appliance for some weeks to allow the joints to settle into their centric position and for the muscles to relax (deprogram).

Once the joints are settled and the muscles relaxed, we either guide the jaw into centered closure or allow it close in the centered position until the first tooth touches.

Following certain bite-adjusting rules, we find this point of first tooth contact and adjust it out of the way. We then locate the next tooth contact in this jaw-centered position and adjust it out of the way; then the next, and the next until all the teeth can hit evenly and properly in this jaw position. In certain situations this occlusal adjustment is first done on study models of your teeth mounted on an articulator (a dental machine that duplicates your bite) to help us plan the procedure.

If we reach a stage where the bite on some teeth is correct, but others do not touch, we build up the bite of the other teeth to the proper level with dental restorations.

If many or most teeth touch correctly to properly support this jaw position, then we may build up "occlusal bite platforms" on the remaining teeth so they share in proper distribution of balanced bite forces. Refinements may be required over time. This is your "home base" for proper support of teeth, muscles and jaw joints, where problems are resolved and we can work. It is where we design and build our dentistry from and where we adjust to.

This is your "centric" position where your joints are properly positioned, your jaw can close correctly, and the teeth bite correctly for proper force distribution. Recent research findings indicate that a balanced bite on natural teeth decreases excess brain activity and can relax excess muscle activation.

For dentistry, this is our Happy Place!

"This is the first time my teeth and jaws have come together right in years. Why haven't other dentists discussed this with me?."

Rick
(After bite adjustment)

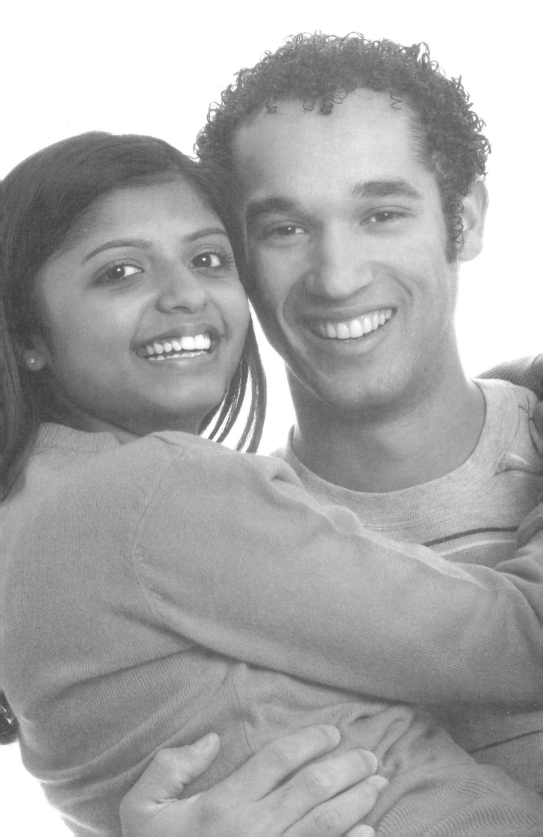

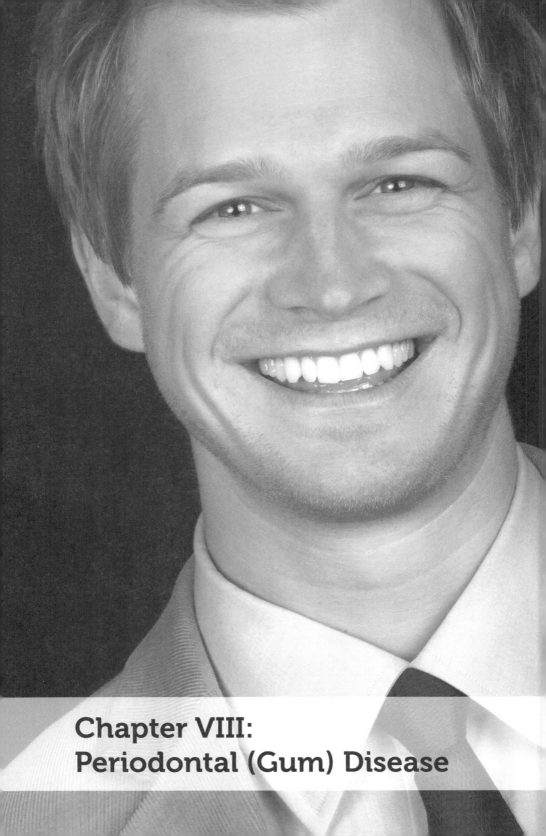

Chapter VIII:
Periodontal (Gum) Disease

What is Gum Disease (Periodontitis)?

Gum disease (periodontal disease, periodontitis, "pyorrhea") is one of man's chronic diseases. In most people over the age of 35, more teeth are lost due to gum disease than to cavities (decay). For most of human history, the average life span was so short that periodontal disease never had time to become a major cause of tooth loss. As we began living longer, periodontal disease became more prevalent, and disease treatment, tooth replacement, fillings, and crowns (dentistry) became part of our culture.

As our life spans increased, periodontal disease became a major problem for us, and mankind began to wonder and study what caused us to become "long in the tooth" as our gums receded. If we live long enough, our rate of cavities (decay) may level off; maintaining our oral health becomes more a matter of preventing and controlling gum disease. Our understanding of the disease has changed, and we now realize that the effects of periodontal disease are not merely confined to tooth loss and destruction of the "gums," but also, outside the mouth, affecting systems and tissues elsewhere in the body.

There is a strong oral-systemic (dental-medical) connection; health or illness in the mouth contributes to health or illness in other body systems. In 1891, Miller published his "Focal Theory of Infection" in which he postulated that dental infections can be the source of infections and disease elsewhere in the body. The idea fell out of favor and was dismissed for over a century. Only now are we realizing how and why Miller was correct. We are truly finding that the infection and inflammation of periodontal (gum) disease cause systemic inflammation and distant body effects. Periodontal disease is a medical problem with a dental solution.

Periodontal disease begins quietly, often with no signs or symptoms. There may be no pain and no indication that the disease is present, with only minor bleeding or soreness when you brush and floss. The disease may silently continue, first causing gingivitis (infection/inflammation of the gums with no underlying damage to the bone). It can then, also silently, cause mild, moderate, and severe periodontitis (loss of the bone and gum tissue which hold and support the teeth).

Gum destruction and tooth loss may be slow or rapid; the disease is often "episodic," occurring in spurts of aggressive destruction between long periods of dormancy. The dental destruction of gum disease, though occasionally apparent in the teen years, often takes many years to become obvious. Over time, one may notice chronic bad breath (halitosis), receding gums (longer teeth), sore or painful gums, and bleeding with brushing or flossing. The gums may show swelling, redness, or draining pus (abscesses), and the teeth may become mobile (loose) and painful. Biting and chewing may cause pain, and the teeth may develop spaces as they move and flare out, with loss of bone support.

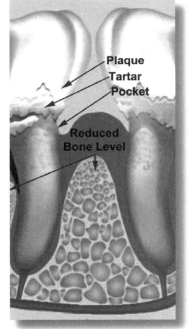

You may see and feel these changes only in the final stages, and then so much bone and gum have been lost that tooth loss is inevitable. The lack of pain often allows us to delude ourselves that no problem exists, and by the time the symptoms develop it may be too late to save the involved teeth.

Illustration courtesy of Dr. Charley Martin, Richmond Smile Center, Richmond, VA.

How Do We Develop Periodontal (Gum) Disease?

As newborn infants, we have few oral bacteria. Once our teeth erupt, bacteria can adhere to the teeth, and the burden of oral bacteria increases as we have more primary (baby) teeth and then as we develop our secondary (adult) teeth. We inherit our oral bacteria from those we kiss and with whom we share food. We usually inherit our first bacteria from our mother with close contact, frequent kisses, and shared food and drink.

Since we tend to inherit our mother's oral bacteria, if she has little decay or gum disease, then our major bacteria will tend to be those that cause little decay or gum disease. If mom (and/or dad) has lots of cavities or bad gums (periodontal disease) then the bacteria we inherit will predispose us to similar problems.

As more and larger teeth erupt, our mouths become colonized by more bacteria; eventually 600-800 different types may call our mouth home. Most of these bacteria are harmless or nearly so; few are outright dangerous to us unless our immune systems become weakened. Many of these bacteria only become harmful when they colonize and become organized into the sticky film we call dental plaque.

Dental plaque is an organized "biofilm" of bacteria, with successive stages of bacteria colonizing this film on the teeth to create an "eco-system" that operates to protect and cultivate the involved bacteria. The bacteria are not easily removed or destroyed, and this self-protecting colony produces more harmful bacteria and more damaging chemicals than could the individual bacterial types alone.

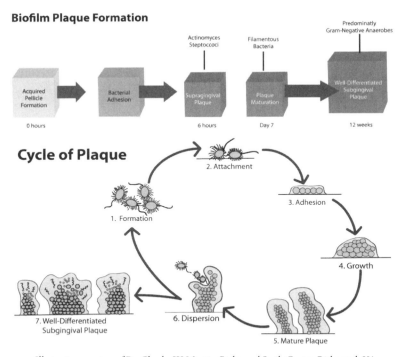

Biofilm Plaque Formation

Illustrations courtesy of Dr. Charles W. Martin, Richmond Smile Center, Richmond, VA.

The bacterial plaque "eco-system" evolves over time and, if not removed, the bacteria evolve from relatively harmless ones to very bad ones. Safe oxygen-loving ("aerobic") bacteria are replaced by more destructive non-oxygen ("anaerobic") ones in the deeper pockets, safe from cleaning and away from oxygen. As the bacteria and the body create deeper pockets in the gums, the bacteria invade more deeply where they have nutrients, warmth, moisture and protection, and become more destructive. The bacteria evolve into a system that has insulating layers and chemicals to protect them from the body's immune system, even while producing chemicals that stimulate the destructive aspects of that immune system. The bacteria, protected in the plaque bio-film, continue to stimulate local bone-destroying inflammation and systemic inflammation causing distant disease. They can also enter the bloodstream through the gums and travel to distant body sites, causing systemic disease.

Dentistry originally thought that the "bad" bacteria became more numerous in this plaque bio-film and that their chemicals, enzymes and by-products caused destruction of the gum tissue and bone. It was further thought that the various stages of mild, moderate, and severe periodontal disease were the result of the bacteria more and more actually invading the gums and bone.

Research now indicates that the major local destruction and systemic effects of periodontal disease begin, not with bacterial invasion of the gums, but with the acids, enzymes, and by-products from these bacteria entering the gums and the body. These bacterial chemicals cause inflammation in the gums and activate the body's immune response which actually attacks the bone and gum, causing the bone to be eaten away by the body's own defenses. The body "sees" the bacterially-infected tooth as diseased and attempts to wall off and shed this diseased tooth and tissue from the gums and jaw bone.

As the body attacks the bad (anaerobic, gram-negative) bacteria, the bacterial breakdown products (endotoxins, Lipopolysaccharides, pathogen-associated molecular patterns) initiate a severe inflammatory response involving cytokine feedback loops and inflammation pathways involving the cytokines (messenger molecules) of inflammation.

The same inflammatory chemical processes which begin in the gums around the diseased teeth, cause the gum disease around the teeth as the body attempts to wall off and shed the diseased tooth and tissue. This same inflammation and bacteria can spread to other body systems, causing disease outside of the mouth.

Gingivitis is the initial stage of gum disease. The gums are reactive, swollen, and inflamed, with no underlying bone destruction yet present; any bacterial pockets in the gums are in soft tissue only. It is easily treated with thorough dental cleaning, good home care, and possibly some additional cleaning aids. If untreated, the disease can progress to more serious periodontal disease and permanent loss of the bone and gum which support the teeth. More severe types of gingival destruction ("Necrotizing Ulcerative Gingivitis") can occur in which we see bacterial invasion and severe destruction of the gum tissue. In most gingivitis, bacteria invasion is limited and the major culprit is the body's immune response stimulated by the plaque bacteria present.

If left untreated and uncleaned, the bacterial plaque biofilm stimulates the body's immune system to actually start resorbing (re-absorbing) the alveolar (tooth-supporting) bone around the teeth, in an attempt to shed the diseased tooth. As bone is resorbed (and the gum tissue swells), the bone may be eaten away to form "pockets" or valleys around the teeth in which bacteria collect. With the bacteria now not accessible with normal tooth-cleaning techniques, more bone is eaten away, pockets are deepened, more bacteria grow, and more bone is lost in a vicious cycle that ends in severe bone loss and the eventual infection, pain, and loss of teeth.

As periodontal disease progresses from gingivitis to mild, moderate, and severe periodontitis, most of the oral destruction is caused by the body's own immune/inflammatory response attacking the bone (and causing distant body effects). Bacteria enter the gums, adding to the destruction, and some bacteria can be found in arterial plaques, arterial thrombi (clots), and abscesses elsewhere in the body.

As periodontitis progresses, bacterial by-products initiate the body's destruction of the periodontal ligament fibers (PDL) holding the teeth in place and of the bone. The bacteria and their by-products are found on tooth roots, in the PDL fibers, in the gum and in the bone. They can enter the bloodstream and initiate the damaging changes noted above.

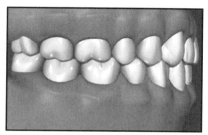

1. Here we see the side view of healthy gums. There is sufficient attached gingiva and there is no recession or inflammation.

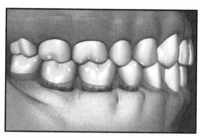

2. If the teeth are not kept properly clean, then there may be formation of 'calculus'. This is a hard substance sometimes called dental stone which is irritating to both the soft (gums) and hard (bone) tissues.

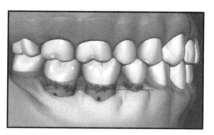

3. In response the gums may recede or inflame. The bone will try to move away from the calculus and therefore recede. This in turn will create deeper pocketing (if the gums do not recede as well) and less bone support of the teeth.

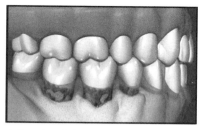

4. If not cleaned, the calculus will continue to accumulate and come closer to the bone.

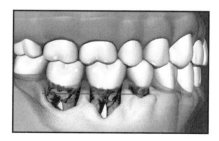

5. The bone in turn recedes more and there is even more bone loss and increased pocketing.

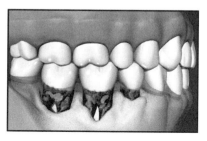

6. The calculus again accumulates and continues the vicious cycle of periodontal disease.

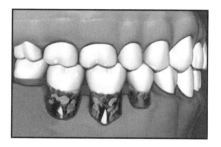

7. Left untreated this results in bad breath, bleeding, red puffy gums and mobile teeth.

Illustrations courtesy of Dr. Charles W. Martin, Richmond Smile Center, Richmond, VA.

As well as localized periodontal destruction, the resultant inflammation and bacterial invasion can contribute to:

- Cardiovascular (atherosclerotic) disease
- Stroke
- Hypertension (high blood pressure)
- Kidney Disease
- Obesity
- Diabetes and Metabolic Syndrome
- Lung Disease
- Alzheimer's Disease and Senile Dementia
- Pregnancy Complications
- Cancer
- Osteoporosis
- Arthritis

Please see our section on The Oral-Systemic Connection (p. 218) for more details, particularly sections A through L.

Gum disease is a disease of bacteria and inflammation that affects both your gums and the rest of your body. It is a silent killer, a medical problem with a dental solution. The bacterial activity and resultant gum (periodontal) inflammation in the mouth can cause bacterial invasion and inflammatory processes resulting in disease elsewhere in the body.

Please see us to avoid the bone destruction, tooth loss, and systemic disease caused by gum disease.

"Dr. Finkel treats you as family. He makes you feel good about your visit. Besides, he's good. I have confidence in his skills. I trust his judgment."

Brenda

Treatment of Periodontal (Gum) Disease

How do we treat gum disease? In the previous section, we noted that periodontal (gum) disease is a disease of the bacterial bio-film that inhabits the teeth and the gums. These bacteria produce chemicals that infiltrate the gums and enter the body. The body's response in attempting to isolate, and get rid of these bacteria and these chemicals, causes the gums to swell with inflammation and causes the bone to be eaten away in an attempt to get rid of, or exfoliate, the teeth and the diseased tissue.

If left untreated and unchecked, gum disease can eventually cause the loss of all the teeth in the mouth as well as pain, discomfort, and dysfunction that naturally result from the loss of your teeth. Proper treatment can save you time, money, discomfort, and loss of confidence. So, how do we treat gum disease and prevent the ongoing damage?

How do we treat early Gum Disease?

If your gum disease is in an early stage, and you are just starting to have minimal infection of the gums around the teeth, then you have gingivitis. Gingivitis is an infection and inflammation of the gums without involvement of the underlying bone. Often, simple cleanings, deep cleanings, or more frequent cleanings can eliminate the problems of gingivitis. Sometimes a deep scaling and root planing (deeper cleaning of the tooth roots with local anesthetic) is required to eliminate the diseased material on the teeth and sometimes just regular cleanings will handle the problem. If the damage to the gums involves more than just the soft tissue, and has started causing the bone to be eaten away, then you have deeper pockets around the teeth in which bacteria can lodge and deeper destruction. In this case, deep scaling and root planing (deeper cleaning of the teeth) is usually necessary to remove the bacteria and eliminate the source of the problem.

We know that if the gum disease is minimal, regular cleanings or more frequent cleanings may handle the problem. If the gum disease has gotten slightly deeper and more involved, you may need a deep scaling and root planing, which is sometimes carried out over several visits to treat the problem.

It has been shown that 3-month cleanings are very beneficial for patients with a history of or active periodontal disease. These 3-month cleanings keep down the bacterial count on the teeth and in the gums. The bacterial count increases rapidly if dental cleanings are more spaced out than 3-month intervals.

How do we treat later (deeper) Gum Disease?

If the periodontal disease has significantly affected the bone, then what you may need is a deeper type of gum treatment in which the gums are gently opened up and moved away from the teeth and the underlying bone is reshaped so that when the gum and bone are allowed to heal, we have eliminated the deep pockets that were reservoirs for bacteria in the gum. Your toothbrush and dental floss are now more effective and can keep you disease-free. These deeper gum treatments are never a cure for the gum disease; if you do not maintain proper hygiene at home, bacteria will re-colonize the gums and teeth and the disease will return. All of our treatments are simply geared to allow the gums to settle and reshape so that your home care becomes effective.

There are additional treatments your dentist may use to help you keep the gums healthy. Placing certain antibiotics in the gum pockets may help reduce the pockets and keep them bacteria-free. Also, certain rinses may be used to keep down the bacterial count in your mouth by acting as local antibiotics without having the normal effect in the body of bacterial resistance that systemic oral antibiotics would have over time.

How do we treat advanced Gum Disease?

In areas of advanced periodontitis where there has been destruction of the bone and the gums surrounding the teeth, your dentist may elect to perform bone ("osseous") grafts, or soft tissue grafts in which the bone and the gum around the teeth can be built up. It is not easy to grow bone around teeth, though specialized techniques have been developed to sometimes accomplish this. Everybody's individual situation is different, so your dentist will need to discuss with you what possibilities exist for restoration of your gums, dental bone, and periodontal health.

In situations where advanced periodontal disease has so ravaged the teeth and the gums that the teeth cannot be saved even with the most sophisticated periodontal repair measures, your options become replacing the teeth with implants, replacing the teeth with bridges, or replacing the teeth with something removable (such as a denture or a partial denture). All these options should be discussed with you as part of a complete and comprehensive dental examination, diagnosis, and treatment planning.

Some notes on Gum Disease and Susceptibility

We inherit different oral bacteria from our parents, spouses, children, and other family members; no two people's bacteria are exactly the same. The degree of decay (cavities) and gum disease we experience are all affected by how well we clean our teeth and gums, the oral bacteria we inherited when we were young, and the additional bacteria we inherited from our spouse. Other factors include our genetic susceptibility to oral disease, the amount of fluoride incorporated into our teeth when we were young, the amount of saliva we have naturally, the buffering or acid-neutralizing capacity of that saliva, the amounts of acid we consume in our drinks, and medications we may take that affect the amount and quality of our saliva. Therefore, we all have different degrees of susceptibility to and resistance to cavities and gum disease. If we maintain proper care of our teeth, with brushing and flossing and avoiding acid-laden drinks, then our response to having cavities or gum disease should be an honest look at what we can do to improve the conditions, but not guilt. Some oral disease factors are outside our control and require a much more complex set of protective strategies.

The overriding goals of comprehensive dentistry should involve looking at all the factors that affect your dental health; cavities, gum disease, bite problems, tooth alignment and the like, and evaluating all the strategies for restoring optimal health and maintaining that oral health over time.

You should expect your dentist to be aware of these many and varied factors, and to evaluate them, discuss them with you, and help you find your individual path to optimal dental health.

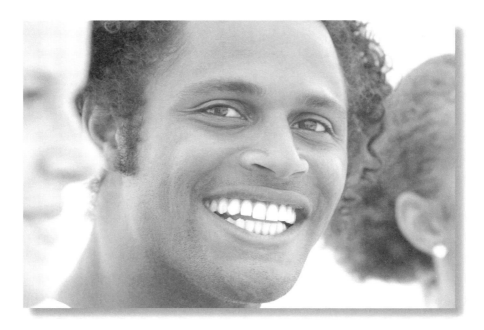

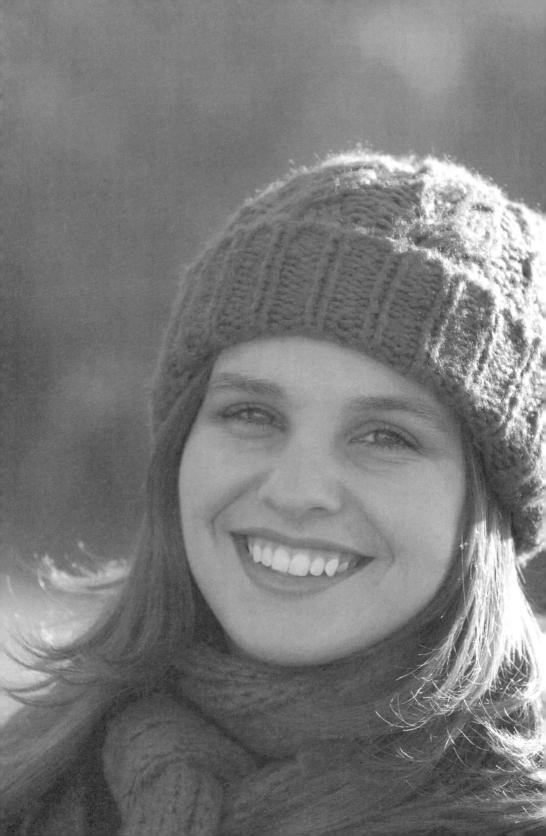

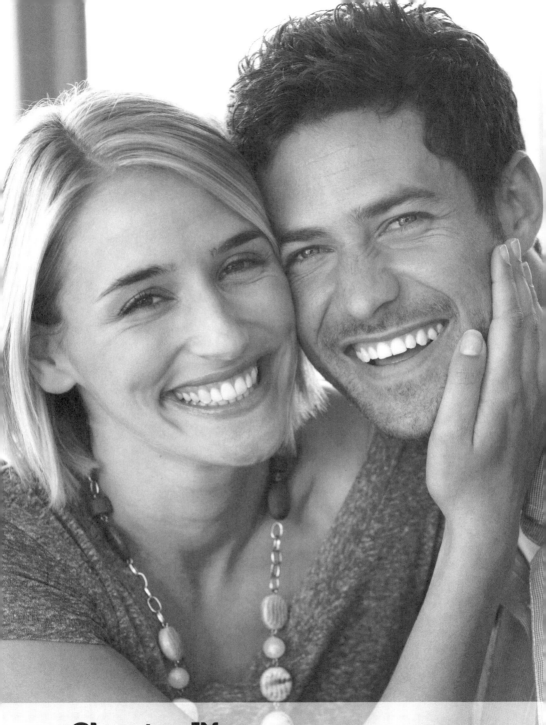

Chapter IX:
Root Canal Therapy

Root Canal Therapy ("Root Canal")

We often hear about "root canals" and how horrible they are. We are conditioned by the media to fear them (as in the movie, "Marathon Man") and to avoid them like the plague. You should not be afraid of root canals, and you should know that they bring about relief of tooth pain and can help you save teeth.

Do Root Canals cause pain?

The mental association of root canal therapy with pain is an interesting one. Root canal therapy is performed to save teeth and relieve pain; but because the already-existing pain is so closely associated in time and space with the root canal procedure, our mind says "root canal = pain." It should be saying "root canal = relief of pain." Where there has been a long-standing tooth abscess, the root canal procedure can temporarily increase the pain, but this is usually very short-term. Any pain after a root canal can usually be handled with a bite adjustment to reduce pressure on the tooth, medications to reduce inflammation and discomfort, steroids to further reduce inflammation-causing chemicals, and, occasionally, antibiotics to handle residual infection.

What exactly is a Root Canal?

Inside a tooth is the pulp tissue that originally formed the tooth in layers from the outside in. As the walls of the tooth are formed and become thicker and stronger, the pulp tissue becomes smaller and smaller until what is left inside the hard tissues of the tooth (enamel, dentin, cementum) is a "pulp chamber" in the crown of the tooth and "pulp canals" in the root(s) of the tooth.

Root Canal Treatment

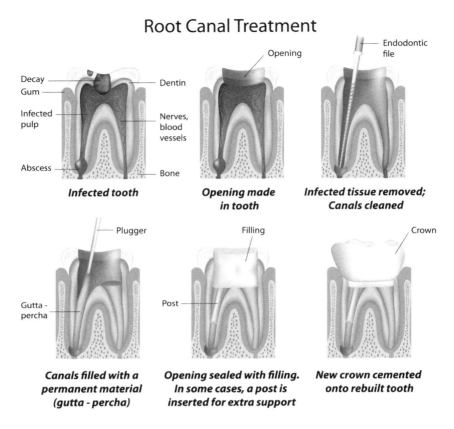

Infected tooth

Labels: Decay, Gum, Infected pulp, Abscess, Dentin, Nerves, blood vessels, Bone

Opening made in tooth

Label: Opening

Infected tissue removed; Canals cleaned

Label: Endodontic file

Canals filled with a permanent material (gutta - percha)

Labels: Plugger, Gutta - percha

Opening sealed with filling. In some cases, a post is inserted for extra support

Labels: Filling, Post

New crown cemented onto rebuilt tooth

Label: Crown

Normally, the tooth structure will remain this way for many years, with the pulp safely enclosed in the crown and roots of the tooth. The pulp chamber and canal(s) will shrink down over time as the pulp forms more tooth structure. Without trauma, disease, or decay (cavity), the pulp will usually continue this way as we age; peacefully and quietly doing its job of forming tooth and sensing changes around it.

Slowly advancing decay in the tooth, normal chewing wear, and normal effects of dental aging will cause the pulp to shrink down at a steady rate. Deep cavities, extreme tooth-grinding, dental treatment, and toothbrush abrasion can cause the pulp to lay down more hard tooth structure (dentin) at an increased rate to "move away" from the irritation and to protect itself.

If decay, extreme wear, and/or acid attack eat away the outside of the tooth faster than the pulp can move away to protect itself, then the pulp is exposed, becomes infected by oral bacteria, and will die.

What are the causes of dental pulp irritation, death, and infection?

1. Deep decay (cavity) eating away the tooth and reaching the pulp so that oral bacteria infect the pulp

2. Trauma to the tooth such as from a fall, baseball accident, fist-fight, or facial injury that can break a tooth root or so move a tooth that the blood vessels entering the root tip (apex) to feed the pulp are severed (disconnected)

3. Extreme grinding wear that causes the dental pulp to recede and finally die

4. A severe crack or split in a tooth that allows the pulp to be traumatized, bacteria to enter, and the pulp to die

5. Periodontal (gum) disease extreme enough for the gum disease bacteria to enter the roots of the tooth and kill the pulp

6. Prior trauma that severs (cuts) the blood vessels to the tooth, so the pulp dies, often leaving a dead, sterile pulp. This can remain asymptomatic (with no pain) for many years and can even form a sterile abscess in which the death-products of the pulp, with no bacterial infection, cause an abscess at the tip of the root. These dead pulps and sterile abscesses can then be infected by bacteria in the blood. Normally, these bacteria are cleared quickly and of no consequence.

7. Idiopathic (of unknown cause) the pulp dies, but with no obvious reason

Of all of the above, deep cavities cause the most infected pulps and dental abscesses.

How does a tooth pulp problem cause an abscess and pain?

Once the dental pulp is infected or dead, bacteria, infection (pus), and destructive chemicals move from the inside of the tooth root out into the bone. Then the infected abscess at the root of the tooth builds up pressure. Unlike an abscess on the arm, which can swell with pressure, this dental abscess is encased in bone and tooth; the pressure builds and pain develops. As the pressure increases, the tooth is elevated in the bone, hits harder when biting, and the pain gets worse.

What is the treatment for an abscessed tooth?

If the tooth is too destroyed by decay and/or gum disease to be successfully treated and restored, then it should be extracted. Extraction performs the two required treatments for any abscess; draining the abscess and removing the source of infection. Extraction of the tooth, though final, does accomplish both.

Ideal treatment involves saving the tooth with root canal therapy, then restoring it to strength and function.

How is Root Canal Therapy ("Root Canal") accomplished?

When a dental (tooth) pulp is diseased, dead, damaged, or otherwise in need of treatment, the dentist first numbs the tooth (local anesthesia or "Novocain"). He or she then isolates the tooth with a "rubber dam" to avoid contamination of the tooth by saliva and prevent swallowing/ aspiration by the patient of dental materials and instruments. Access into the pulp is accomplished by preparing a hole in the top of the tooth and carefully extending that preparation until the pulp is exposed. The preparation is then extended until the pulp chamber is "unroofed" and access is available to all parts of the pulp chamber and root (pulp) canals.

The pulp chamber is cleaned, and the canals filed, enlarged and shaped with various instruments. All areas of the pulp chamber and roots are then cleaned and sterilized with various irrigation solutions, which dissolve necrotic (dead) tissue and kill bacteria.

The canals are carefully shaped just to, but still inside of, the root tips (apices) with special files. The working length, to just inside the root tip (apex), is determined with electronic apex locators, x-rays, and paper points that detect the location of moisture just past the root tip.

The root canals (pulp canals) are carefully confirmed for length, size, and shape. They are then dried and filled with a filling material (like gutta-percha, a relative of latex also used inside golf balls) and a special sealer. The filling material and sealer seal up the inside of the tooth to prevent future infection or re-infection.

In Root Canals, are the tooth roots removed?

No. Root canal therapy is performed inside the roots of the tooth. Only in special circumstances, with special procedures, is a root removed. This is not a part of regular root canal therapy.

Does all the Root Canal filling material stay inside the root?

Ideally, the root canal is measured, shaped, and sealed to just inside the root tip. Some filling materials or sealer may be extruded past the root tip but is usually of no consequence. It is better for the root canal to be well-cleaned and well-sealed, even if just past the root tip, than to be under-cleaned or under-sealed.

What now for the tooth?

The tooth must now be sealed and restored with a filling ("core") and usually a crown. Root canal teeth have often lost a lot of tooth structure from decay or trauma. Preservation of tooth structure and restoration of function are critical; usually a core and crown are necessary to accomplish this.

Above all else, the tooth must be sealed so that the top of the root canal is sealed off from the saliva and bacteria of the mouth. More than from any other cause, properly done root-canal teeth are lost from loss of this seal, with re-decay, and re-contamination of the root canal.

Failure to restore the tooth can also cause loss of the weakened tooth when it breaks or splits from not having been restored with a needed crown.

Are all Root Canals successful?

No. Poorly done root canals do not eliminate all of the infection and, thus, do not prevent later re-infection. If a tooth is cracked or split, then it will be lost in spite of an excellent root canal. There can be hidden microscopic channels in the root canal system of the tooth, so that even a well-done root canal may fail.

If my Root Canal fails, what are my options?

If a root canal fails, then the first option is to retreat (redo) the root canal. Secondly, the dentist and patient may elect to surgically clean out and seal the tip of the root, accessing through the gum and bone, in a process known as an apico-ectomy. Thirdly, the tooth may require extraction and replacement with a bridge or implant.

A final thought on Root Canals

Root canals usually relieve pain, are highly successful, and help maintain teeth that would otherwise be lost. The tooth then requires proper restoration to maintain a good seal, provide strength, and restore function.

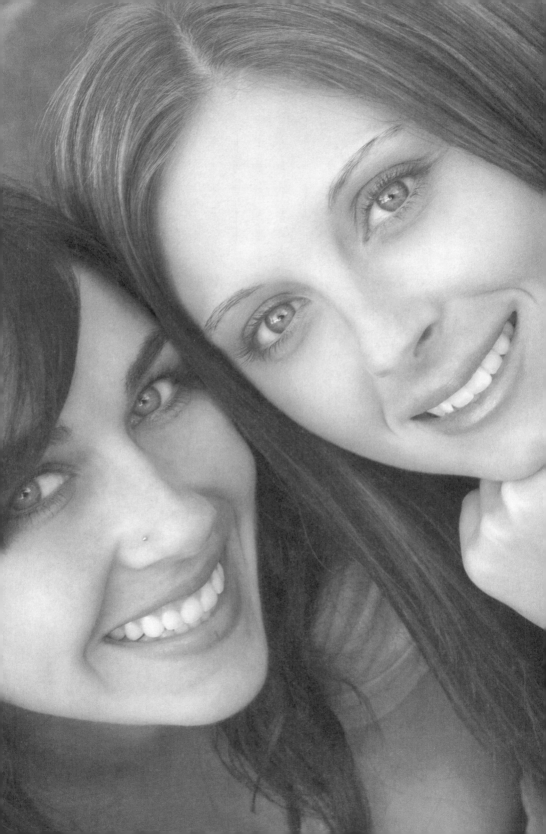

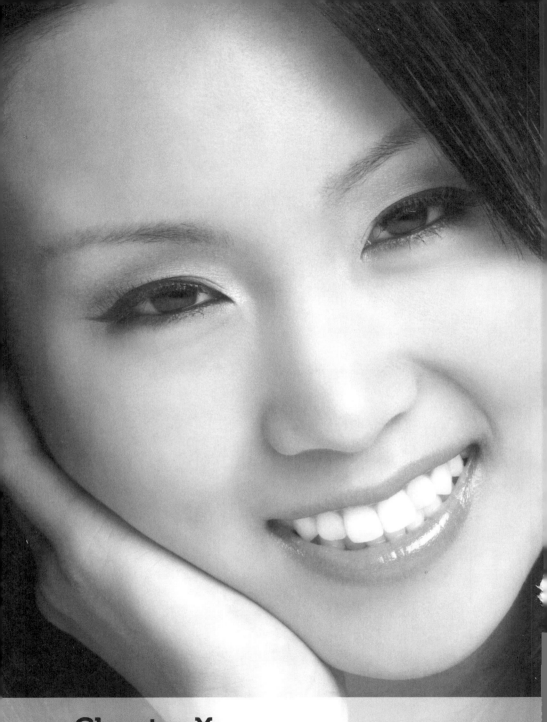

Chapter X:
Dental Implants

What are Dental Implants?

Dental implants are titanium or titanium alloy cylinders (root forms) which are surgically implanted into the bone of the jaw and which are then used, like tooth roots, to support crowns or dental restorations above them; just as a tooth root supports the tooth crown above it.

Dental implants represent one of the greatest innovations in oral health and dentistry since dentistry evolved as a healing art. In modern dentistry they are the most effective, and ultimately most conservative, way in which a missing tooth can be replaced while maintaining normal dental forces on the other teeth and avoiding destructive treatment of adjacent teeth.

Let's Begin with Basics:

What is the history of Dental Implants?

Implants were attempted as far back as the Mayan civilization, and possibly earlier, as a way to replace missing teeth. Pieces of shell, gold teeth, parts of bone, ivory, metal screws, and even other people's teeth were implanted in the sockets of extracted teeth to act as replacements. The first modern-age dental implants of the 1960's and 1970's were "blade" implants or "sub-periosteal" implants and did not use today's materials.

With the former, blade implants, the part of the implant in the bone was in the form of a narrow strip or plate of metal and ran some distance in the jawbone. Part of the implant then rose out of the bone, through the gum tissue, to form a post on which the tooth or teeth were built. The sub-periosteal implant was designed as a framework that fit intimately on the surface of the bone of the upper or lower jaw and was held in place by the overlying gum tissue binding down the framework to the bone surface. Posts extended through the gum into the mouth; onto these posts the teeth would be built. These first modern age dental implants were made of various surgical steels, thought to be very durable and strong; they were tolerated by the body but not truly accepted as part of it, and they failed.

What is a modern Dental Implant?

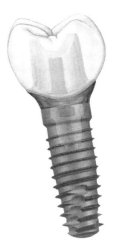

Modern dental implants have mainly evolved into "root-form" implants; cylinders of titanium or titanium alloy roughly the size and general shape of tooth roots. Titanium has been found to be a strong, durable metal to which the bone can fuse (osseointegrate), and the gum tissue can attach. The surface of modern dental implants is threaded, textured and otherwise prepared so the bone can best form to and fuse to it. The current size and cylindrical form of most dental implants allow them to fit into the jawbone (upper and lower) for the replacement of missing teeth in harmony with the position and form of the other teeth and tooth roots.

A dental implant abutment (connecting element) is then attached to the dental implant, exiting through the gum and into the mouth. Onto this implant abutment, the new tooth crown or restoration is built.

The modern implant system consists of three parts; the Implant itself, the Dental Implant Abutment (with seating screw), and the Crown (or other dental restoration) that is seated on the abutment. Some modern dental implant systems have the implant and abutment as a single unit.

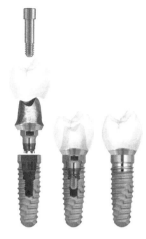

When the abutment is held onto the implant with a special seating screw and the crown restoration is cemented to the implant abutment, this is referred to as a cement-retained (or cemented) implant restoration. For some special-needs situations, the crown and abutment are made as one unit and, as a single unit, screwed onto the implant body. This is a screw-retained implant restoration. When the implant and abutment are a single unit, then crown or over-lying restoration is cement-retained.

Research is currently being done on implants made of zirconia and of titanium-zirconia alloy. While promising, as of this printing, research has not yet established that these new implant materials are as durable, as workable, or as well-accepted by the body as those in current use.

What is a Dental Implant abutment?

Most modern dental implant systems allow the Implant (implant "body") to be placed in the bone, an abutment to be attached with a seating screw, and the crown (or other restoration) to be seated on the abutment. Implant abutments come in many designs, shapes, angles, and materials. The abutment design is matched to the implant body to which it is or will be attached.

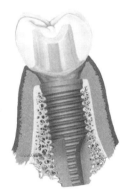

The abutment shape is matched to the implant, the gum (height and thickness) which it goes through to emerge into the mouth, and the form needed to support the gums and the dental restoration. The abutment angle allows the crown angle to properly align with other teeth in the mouth and can often correct for difficulties encountered in the original implant surgical placement. The abutment material is usually zirconia or metal; zircona being strong and more esthetically-colored (tooth-like), metal being even stronger and needed in high-stress situations. Some implant systems make the abutment an extension of the implant body; the unit being entirely metal.

What is the difference between a natural tooth and a Dental Implant?

While previous implant materials and shapes were allowed and tolerated by the body, current implants allow the human body to heal to them and accept the implants more as a part of the body. Important in force distribution is the fact that natural teeth are suspended in the jawbone by millions of fibers, the PDL or "Periodontal Ligament," so the natural tooth is not fused to the bone, but held in place by this network of fibers so that there is space and cushion to act as a shock absorber, and the natural tooth has room to move before it must actually contact and compress the bone around it. This shock-absorber effect is what allows natural teeth to absorb biting forces without cracking and shattering.

The dental implant has no such supporting fiber network; the implant body is fused directly to the bone with no intervening shock-absorbing network. Because of this, the bite ("occlusion") on the implant must be more carefully designed and regulated, and must be somewhat different from those forces on natural teeth. Without the shock-absorber effect being available to implants, if an implant is over-stressed, the results can be loss (or "die-back") of the bone around the implant, fracture of the implant, fracture of the overlying crown or crowns, and loosening or fracture of the screw holding the implant and crown abutment together. The dentist must properly design the bite and function on the implants to avoid such problems.

The importance of dental bone for teeth and Dental Implants:

When a tooth is present, it stimulates the bone to grow and maintain around it. The forces of chewing and normal use act on the fibers holding the tooth in the jaw bone; these forces of tension pull on the fibers and stimulate bone growth, mineralization of the bone matrix, angiogenesis (development of blood vessels), and laying down of the normal bone structure. The continued stimulation of the bone by the presence and function of the tooth maintains presence and health of the bone.

When a tooth or multiple teeth are lost, the jaw bone surrounding and supporting the tooth or teeth is lost. It immediately begins to collapse in thickness and height into the area once occupied by the tooth root(s). Because the stimulating effect of the now-missing tooth is no longer present, the body "sees" no reason to maintain the bone. The physiologic factors which once caused the bone to develop and maintain no longer exist, and the body starts re-absorbing the bone structure. The height of the bone around the missing tooth begins to decrease, and the volume of the bone which once supported the tooth (root) so rapidly diminishes that 60% of the total bone volume may be lost in six months. The maintenance of this local bone is important for support of the adjacent teeth, proper gum structure, esthetics, and the future ability to place an implant to restore the missing tooth. We like to keep the bone!

The bottom line is: if you take out the tooth, the bone goes away. Said differently: if you lose the tooth, you lose the bone. Once lost, the bone is not easy to re-grow; it can be done, but involves additional treatment (bone grafting) and additional cost. Maintenance of this important bone after tooth extraction is termed site (or socket) preservation and should ideally happen at the time of tooth extraction if an implant is not placed immediately. Today, most implants are placed at the time of tooth extraction to minimize bone loss, shorten treatment time, and decrease cost.

Site preservation: saving bone for Dental Implants:

Our goal is to preserve bone health and volume for immediate implant placement, or future implant placement after healing has occurred; ie. site preservation.

Site (or socket) preservation involves first insuring that the tooth extraction site is disease-free. If the tooth has an infection or abscess present, this may require antibiotics for some days prior to the extraction or a larger dose of antibiotics immediately prior to the extraction. It certainly includes careful and complete cleaning out (curettage, debridement) of the extraction site once the tooth is removed to make certain that all bacterial contamination of the site has been eliminated.

Into this site, we place bone graft material (freeze-dried bone or demineralized freeze-dried bone) which has been chemically and/or radiation treated to insure its safety for use. We then place a tissue-fiber (collagen) membrane over the bone graft in a single or double layer, suture the area, and often cover it with a tissue-compatible sealing material. When practical, natural gum tissue is moved or grafted to cover the bone graft. In some cases, donor grafting gum tissue may be used to cover and build up the area. Bone Morphogenic Proteins (BMP), blood derived proteins, or other molecular growth factors may be used to enhance bone formation and healing.

In areas of tooth extraction or prior tooth loss in the same area, more involved bone grafting with special membranes, larger amounts of bone, blocks of bone, and gum tissue replacement may be involved. The tooth extraction area may be grafted and structured to accept implant(s) immediately or it may be prepared and structured so that an implant can be successfully placed after healing has occurred. Again, the important thing is the maintenance and/or creation of adequate bone and gum tissue to maintain the health of the bone for the adjacent teeth, and adequate support for implants to be placed immediately or in the future.

Surgical placement of the Dental Implant:

A dental implant can be placed immediately upon extraction of the tooth, within a short time, or years after the tooth was extracted. The best bone support and best long-term results are obtained when the largest volume of bone is present. This is usually the case at time of extraction, shortly there-after, or when bone grafting has been performed. See the above section on site (socket) preservation (p. 118). The earlier your implant treatment is begun, the more and easier are your options.

Timing options handled, (your dental extraction being in the past or present), the surgeon will place your dental implant into bone, below and inside the gum, along with any needed bone graft, membranes, additional gum grafts, biologic healing factors, and sutures as indicated. The implant will be left either totally covered by the gum or connected to a healing abutment showing through the gum so the gum can heal around it. Implants placed into the upper jaw may require "sinus-lift" procedures to elevate the sinus floor with bone grafting to give enough bone height for implant placement.

All of these options will be discussed by your surgeon beforehand, and even though scary-sounding, are usually completed with relatively little discomfort and few complications. Sedation is usually available for the surgical procedure if requested.

Implant healing time prior to restoration:

The implant is then usually left to heal undisturbed for two to four months or more before tooth restoration, as determined by your dental surgeon. It usually takes at least two to three months in the lower jaw and three to four months in the upper jaw for the implant to "heal in" or osseointegrate. The bone in the lower jaw is more solid, so the implants are able to be restored or "loaded," sooner. In the upper jaw, the bone is less dense, sinus elevation procedures (see above) may be needed, and it usually takes the longer healing time of three to four months for the bone to solidify and the implant to osseointegrate. Upper or lower, once healing has occurred, the implant or implants are ready to build upon (restore). During healing, the implants must be allowed to heal (osseointegrate) without movement. Micro-movement during the healing phase reduces bone healing around the implant and may cause implant failure. Macro-movement or micro-movement of the implant must be avoided during the healing phase.

Proper healing is confirmed by tissue form, comfort, ability of the implant to comfortably accept turning (torqueing) pressure and proper "sounding" of the implant by a special instrument that checks proper sound response to tapping on the implant.

What is immediate temporization ("load") of Implants?

Immediate "loading" of an implant means placing a tooth on the implant (or teeth on implants) on the day of implant placement. Generally, this new tooth must be properly protected so no forces from chewing or biting are placed on it; so no movement of the healing implant can occur. The safest techniques are those that allow no forces on, and no possible movement of, the implant during healing.

What is the success rate for Dental Implants?

Dental implants, properly placed, allowed to heal correctly, properly loaded (dentally restored), and properly maintained – show a 95-98% success rate. Proper surgical technique, a safe healing period, and correctly engineered dentistry on the implants maximize success and should not be hurried or minimized. Most problems with implants occur within the first year and can be treated with localized therapy or implant replacement, often at little or no cost to you.

What do I do for a temporary tooth while my extraction and Implant heal?

After extraction, surgical grafting, implant placement and during healing, there may be a period of time before your final tooth replacement can be made and seated on your implant(s). For a back tooth which does not show, often no temporary replacement is necessary and simply leaving it alone is your easiest, least expensive, alternative.

If your missing tooth is a front tooth or one that shows, most people want a temporary replacement for esthetic reasons and to avoid social embarrassment.

Possible temporary replacements are:

1. An "Essix" retainer in which your natural tooth crown or a denture tooth is held in place in a clear retainer so the tooth still appears to be in place; it is removed for chewing hard foods and for sleeping.

2. A "flipper" partial denture; an acrylic partial denture that fits to your other teeth and holds one or more teeth to replace the missing one(s). Stronger than an Essix retainer, this is better for eating (still soft foods) and social occasions.

3. A bonded tooth; bonded to the adjacent teeth; removed and rebonded as treatment proceeds. This option usually costs slightly more than the flipper partial and is more secure.

4. A temporary bridge may be used as your temporary tooth replacement if the adjacent teeth are scheduled to receive crowns or veneers. This is often the most secure, allows preview of the esthetics of your final teeth, and allows your dentist to establish desired size, length, form, function, and esthetics of your final dental restoration. The cost is usually greater, and may be incorporated into your overall dental rehabilitation fee.

5. Immediate temporization of the implant with a provisional crown. This will hold the space and restore esthetics, but not touch opposing teeth in bite or function, so there are no forces on the implant during healing.

What dental restorations are available on my Implant(s)?

Depending on your individual situation, there are many implant restoration possibilities, including:

1. Single missing tooth: Single implant: usually restored with an abutment and crown.

2. Multiple missing teeth: Multiple implants/abutments/crowns: one for each tooth, or multiple spaced implants to replace alternating teeth; then crowns and bridges.

3. Full-arch missing teeth: Implants/abutments/crowns for each missing tooth.

4. Full-arch missing teeth: Implants/to replace every other tooth root, then a full-arch (roundhouse) bridge or separate bridges.

5. Full arch: Denture which snaps to a "locator" attachment on each implant.

6. Bar-retained overdenture: a CAD-CAM (machined) bar is attached to and stabilizes the implants. A full denture snaps onto the bar and is held securely in place.

7. Full arch: Denture/Hybrid appliance with metal framework and acrylic teeth, locked in place on your implants.

8. Full arch: Bridge framework with porcelain and gold teeth fused to the bridge framework, locked in place on your implants.

Why restore a missing tooth?

Bite collapse, TMJ/muscle problems, esthetics:

Missing front teeth are usually replaced for cosmetic and esthetic reasons: No-one wants to be seen with the gap from a missing tooth. Our society expects a good looking, well-maintained smile; implants are often the most conservative technique for restoring your smile.

What about back teeth? Why replace or restore a missing back tooth? After all, it may not be seen if we don't open really wide or if nobody is looking.

Why restore back teeth?

1. A missing back tooth decreases our ability to chew; biting forces are increased on the remaining teeth and often onto the other side. Over-stressed remaining teeth can break and fail.

2. A missing back tooth leaves a gap; into this gap fall (lean) the adjacent teeth and the opposing tooth (its would-be biting tooth). The adjacent teeth, now leaning into the space, become more prone to gum disease and cavities. The opposing tooth grows into the space (upper "super-erupting" down or lower "super-erupting" up) and can be lost as it "grows" out of the bone.

3. The back teeth, now having shifted sideways, up, and down, no longer hit evenly and together. They bang into each other forcefully and can break and split.

4. Even if (especially if) these now mal-positioned teeth are not lost, their uneven bite causes trauma to the TMJs (jaw joints) and excess spasm in the biting muscles.

5. The dental results are more gum disease, cavities, and broken teeth. The facial results are head, neck, and face pain; also pain and dysfunction of the jaw joints ("TMJ").

6. Esthetically, loss of back teeth and the resultant "bite collapse" cause excess pressure on the front teeth. The front teeth, with all this excess pressure and force, can now flare outward, develop spacing, weaken, fail, and be lost.

All of this dental failure can begin with the loss of a single back tooth. That is why we restore and replace a missing back tooth; often with an implant for the most sound and conservative result. Recent research indicates that a balanced bite increases normal brain activity in the areas of working memory and cognitive function (Franco, Al., et al., Brazil), lessening the effects of aging, stress, and brain degeneration (Narita, N., et al. and Miyamoto, I., et al.).

Why get an Implant?
Why not a Bridge or Partial Denture?

Of all dental tooth replacements, the implant-supported restoration is most like your natural teeth for comfort, stability, and support. Also, by preparing (cutting down) healthy adjacent teeth for crowns to hold a bridge, you are turning a one-tooth problem into a three-or-more-tooth problem. That is, one missing tooth needing treatment becomes more teeth being treated as two or more adjacent teeth are prepared (cut down) for crowns (damaged).

The average crown lasts 8-12 years before some additional treatment is needed. The crown may fail due to re-decay (cavity), fracture, or root canal problems. A bridge, with two or more end (abutment) crowns has an increased possibility of problems or failure, so you can expect a bridge to require more replacement over time.

Implants have been shown to have a much longer life span. By placing an implant with abutment and crown, rather than a bridge, to replace a missing tooth, you usually:

a) Save the adjacent teeth from additional damage

b) Protect the adjacent teeth by better distributing chewing and biting forces

c) Save the adjacent teeth from future dental treatment involving additional risk and cost

d) Save money over your lifetime with one implant + abutment + crown rather than multiple replacement bridges or other dental treatments over the years

Implants more cost-effectively restore normal chewing efficiency, bite support, esthetics, and phonetics. Current research indicates that implant-supported restorations improve brain function in the areas of touch, sensation, and chewing efficiency.

How long can I wait after tooth extraction to do my Implants?

It is crucial to remember that the longer you wait to replace a missing tooth, the more the bone of the jaw and face will decrease. Early planning and treatment increase the odds of functional and esthetic success with lower cost. Bone and tissue grafting can help; the sooner the better!

Can Implants help with a difficult denture?

Yes, implants can stabilize a full or partial denture to make chewing and speaking easier.

Upper dentures are often quite satisfactory without any implants, so an upper complete denture may be all you need if you have lost your upper teeth, though bone loss over time can lessen the ease and comfort of your upper denture. If you cannot tolerate the palate (central part on the roof of the mouth) of the upper denture, then a palate-less denture can be made which is supported on five or six upper implants. This appliance can snap to place and be removable or fixed in place.

The lower denture often presents the greatest problems for the patient:

Compared to the upper jaw, there is less lower jaw tissue support, and the lower bone becomes reduced and sharper. The lower gum tissue is thinner and more delicate, and the tongue, lips, and cheeks all tend to lift and move the lower denture; so it is almost never as satisfactory and stable as the upper.

A lower denture can be:

1. Retained with two implants and "locator-type" attachments which allow it to be snapped in place to hold more securely (an "Implant-retained" denture)

2. Retained and supported with four or five implants and "locator-type" attachments which allow it to be snapped in place and stabilized much more securely for chewing and function; also removable but much more secure (an "Implant-supported" denture)

3. Replaced with a "bar" denture in which the implants are attached to each other with a metal bar, and the denture clips to this bar for security and stability

4. Replaced with five to six implants and a fixed dental appliance comprised of a metal framework and processed acrylic/composite teeth. This is a "hybrid" appliance, fixed in place on the implants. It is very secure and comfortable, may require extra diligence in cleaning, and may require reprocessing or replacement of the teeth after some years

5. Replaced with multiple implants, with fixed porcelain-to-metal framework or multiple implants/abutments with cemented crowns and bridges. These two options represent the Mercedes-Benz of options for comfort, function, and esthetics, and come at increased technical involvement and cost

All options should be explored, as you are choosing treatments for your lifetime that affect your ongoing comfort and confidence, taking into account your specific needs, wants, and budgetary concerns.

Can I be allergic to the titanium of the Implants?

This is theoretically possible, but we have not seen such a case.

What about Mini-Implants?

These are available and a reasonable alternative when cost is a major factor, when you still need a denture stabilized, especially an existing denture you do not want to replace. However, options, longevity, and success remain greater with regular implants.

Can Implants help with orthodontics?

Yes…Implants can act as anchor teeth for orthodontic correction of the other teeth. Orthodontics can be planned so the implants may be placed prior to the orthodontics to help with tooth movement, if we can project the required final implant location relative to the final orthodontic result. Implants may also be placed after orthodontics are completed and final tooth spacing for the implant(s) has been finalized.

If I lose more teeth, can I have more Implants?

Yes; you should always receive a full diagnosis and treatment plan so other teeth with questionable prognosis can be planned for. Your treatment should always allow for future loss of these teeth, additional possible implants, and incorporation of your existing dentistry into a new phase of oral rehabilitation.

What Now?

This has been an introduction to the exciting world of modern implant dentistry. Please ask us to explore options pertaining to your individual circumstances and needs, so we can establish a treatment plan and help you maintain that smile you have always wanted.

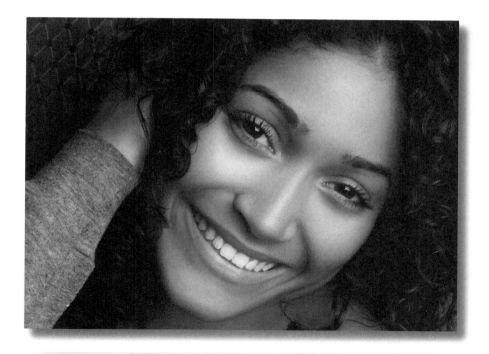

"I've been a patient of Dr. Finkel since 1994. My wife and I entrust our entire family's dental health to Dr. Finkel and his staff.

"Over the years we've had nothing short of superb quality care that is always done in a professional manner We would highly recommend Dr. Finkel's office to anyone."

Tab

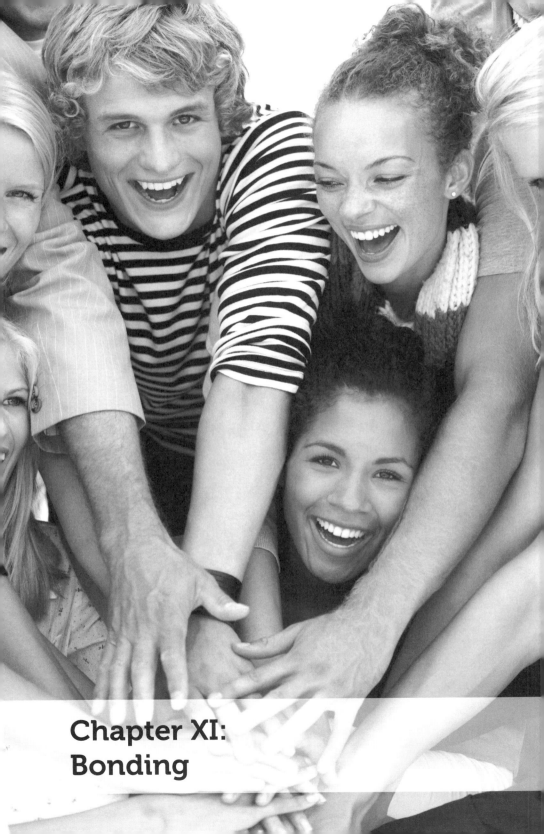

Chapter XI:
Bonding

Composite Bonding

Bonding refers to the attaching of tooth-like, enamel-colored materials to the teeth. Though technically the term refers to any of the techniques used to make dental materials adhere to (stick to) the teeth, for our usage, bonding will be used to mean attaching composite (resin) tooth-like filling material to the tooth for fillings, tooth rebuilding, and dental cosmetics on the front teeth.

Bonding is the term used for attaching porcelain veneers, crowns, and other dental additions to teeth by chemical means. Here, we will use it to mean those times when composite (tooth rebuilding) material is the final restorative material.

Bonding uses both chemical-curing (self-curing, cures after mixing) or light-curing materials (worked in place and then set-up, fixed, by light activation). For most current bonding techniques, we employ the light-curing methods, as they let us work longer with the materials prior to set, achieve stronger and more durable curing of the material, and result in a more color-stable and esthetic result over time.

What is the Bonding Process?

So, for our purposes: Bonding means building up of front or back teeth for fillings and veneers with a material we can work and sculpt to the form we want in the mouth and then using a special light-emitting "gun" to cure (set) the material to its final shape and form.

The treatment steps involved are; visualization of the desired result, tooth preparation, bonding/adhesive steps, placing and forming the material, light-curing the material, then finishing, adjusting and polishing it.

What are the Advantages of Bonding?

Most older dental materials did not adhere (bond) to teeth, so crowns and filling materials were held in the tooth with retentive shapes, undercuts and grooves cut in the tooth to hold in fillings, or retentive shapes on crown preparations so cements could harden in a crown and mechanically lock it onto the tooth.

In recent decades, techniques were developed to allow dental materials to actually bond (adhere) to tooth structure by chemical and "micro-mechanical" means. Since we can now bond to the tooth, we can add material, rather than cutting tooth away to lock restorations on or in teeth.

We can now add to teeth rather than take away; dentistry has become additive, not subtractive, and can keep teeth more whole.

Why Do Bonding?

With bonding, we can preserve tooth structure with less damage to healthy teeth. Biting forces must be balanced because the bonding is sometimes not as strong as crowns but is a good thing to keep teeth more whole.

For front teeth, veneers can be completed with bonded composite material, with less need for reducing teeth as with porcelain veneers. Small gaps, chips, and discolored spots can be covered, filled, and hidden at lower cost and with greater ease. These composite veneers and composite fillings are very esthetic and preserve tooth. For back teeth, fillings can be bonded-in with less cutting into the tooth, thereby preserving healthy tooth structure.

Why Have Bonded Fillings?

Properly prepared and bonded "composite" (tooth colored) fillings take significantly more time and skill to perform properly and so should cost more than the older silver fillings. Many extra steps, better isolation, and more exacting techniques are required to properly do a bonded composite filling so it functions well, looks good, is comfortable, and has longevity. Please expect this extra care when you elect these bonded fillings.

When properly done, these bonded fillings have the advantage of strengthening the tooth. Older fillings were mechanically "locked into" the tooth but did nothing to strengthen it. Bonded fillings can actually bond to the walls of the tooth, help hold it together, and increase its strength and resistance to fracture. When a crown is indicated for strength in repairing a tooth but cannot be done for time or financial reasons, a bonded filling may help hold the tooth together until a crown can be done.

Bonding can also be done on back teeth, the inside of (upper) front teeth, and the front edges of lower front teeth to build up the bite for proper jaw support. Again, we are adding to, not taking away, tooth structure. More conservative than veneers and crowns, bonding can eliminate spaces, gaps, and defects in the front teeth to mimic nature's beauty at lower cost.

Remember, often the best dentistry is less dentistry or no dentistry; preserving healthy tooth structure. Conservative dental bonding can help preserve your dental health, support your bite, and fix dental problems; all while helping to give you that smile you have always wanted.

"Dr. Finkel and his staff rock!"   *Monica*

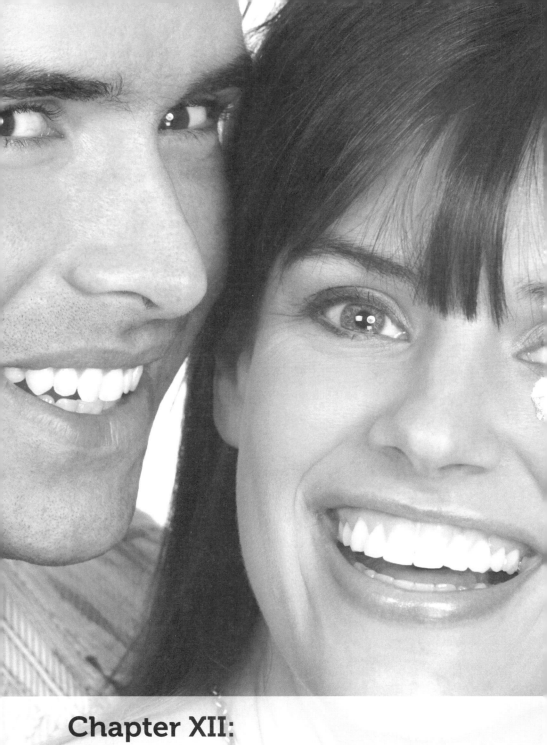

Chapter XII:
Veneers

Veneers
(Porcelain Laminate Veneers)

Veneers ("Porcelain Veneers" or "Bonded Veneers") are one of modern dentistry's marvels; these thin tooth-shaped pieces of porcelain can be bonded to teeth to give you a dazzling beautiful smile without excessive reduction ("preparation") of the teeth. They are a smile-making miracle and can change your life, quickly giving you that smile you have always wanted; but they still come with some warnings and cautions.

A dentist should always place the welfare of his patient above all else; above personal gain, above profit, above feel-good notoriety. Your dentist should always strive to give you the smile, chewing ability, dental health, and comfort you desire with the least amount of tooth preparation and lost tooth enamel. Your dentist should work to keep your teeth as whole as possible while helping you attain your dental goals.

Many patients have been disappointed in the look of their natural teeth, and unhappy with the smile those teeth represent. They have heard that porcelain veneers can give them an instant Hollywood smile; this becomes their dream and their goal. What they don't know is that while veneers are wonderful, they may not be permanent; they may not be "forever."

Porcelain veneers, when bonded to tooth enamel become very strong. They bond most strongly and durably to the outer tooth layer, enamel, and less durably to the inner tooth layer, dentin. Bonds to enamel are much more long lasting than those to dentin; the more enamel left on the tooth, the better the bond and the longer your veneer will likely last. If your teeth have had prior dentistry, or are broken down and fractured, the odds are greater that less enamel remains, more of the bonding will be to tooth dentin, and that the veneer can weaken over time.

"Prep-less veneers" or "minimal-prep veneers" strive to minimally prepare teeth for veneers to be made and bonded, leaving as much enamel as possible for a strong, long-lasting bond and a strong long-lasting veneer. If the tooth is too broken or damaged, then a crown-veneer will give greater strength and longevity.

Veneers can fail in certain ways:

1. As they age, the bond to the tooth weakens, especially if less enamel remained on the original tooth; all bonding weakens with time. Over time, this weakened bond causes the veneer to be less re-inforced and possibly fracture. It can also "debond" or separate from the tooth.

2. Over time the porcelain veneer can chip and break from biting and chewing forces, thus leading to the need for repair.

3. Over time, biting and chewing forces can cause the tooth to flex and bend more than does the porcelain veneer. The bonded veneer can then separate ("debond"), break, or lose seal at the edges.

4. Over time, thermocycling (temperature changes from food and drink) can cause weakening of the material bonding the veneer to the tooth.

5. Flexing (#3 above) and thermocycling (#4 above) can result in staining and cavity (decay) at the veneer edges.

All these failure modes can be minimized with proper tooth preparation (leaving as much enamel as possible), proper tooth design, veneer design, and proper bonding techniques. Proper bite adjustment (see the section on bite adjustments, p. 84), proper home care, and use of a nightguard to minimize destructive bite forces can also help ensure longevity of your veneers.

Alternatives to Veneers

- Orthodontics (braces) can correct a crooked smile, crooked teeth, and spaces. Braces can also reposition your teeth to minimize the extent or number of veneers necessary to complete your smile. Braces can redistribute (even-up) spaces between teeth, so minimal veneers or bonding can be used to close the remaining spaces at lower cost and less tooth preparation.

- Recontouring (smoothing) tooth edges can remove jagged points to give a straighter, more even smile line, and tooth recontouring can bring teeth physically and visually back in line for a more even and natural smile.

- Bonding (bonding on of tooth-enamel-like material) can close spaces (gaps), recontour teeth, or fill in incisal edges with little or no tooth reduction to keep the teeth as whole as possible.

- Whitening, or Bleaching, can make teeth lighter and more dazzling with no tooth reduction or enamel loss. Many techniques are available, and we will be happy to review them with you.

- Gingival (Gum) Recontouring can make the teeth look longer, fuller, and more natural; it can also reduce the look of a "gummy" smile where too much gum shows when you smile.

These alternatives to veneers are more conservative ways to improve your smile, with less cost, less treatment, and less removal of natural tooth structure. The more natural tooth structure you leave, the healthier and more long-lasting the teeth. Often, the best dentistry is less dentistry or no dentistry.

Now, for Veneers:

Assuming that you want to really improve your smile, none of the veneer-alternatives appeal to you, and your teeth can accept porcelain veneers or porcelain veneer-crowns, what do you need to know before you proceed with dental porcelain veneers?

First, porcelain veneers are thin porcelain shells bonded to teeth to improve their looks. They are bonded with chemicals and materials that form a layer bonded to the tooth and to the veneer to seal and hold the veneer in place. The bonding process actually increases the strength of the veneer so it is more durable and longer-lasting. Your dentist should use a meticulous technique, to plan, model, prepare, impress, temporize, bond, and finish your veneers.

You should practice excellent home care, (cleaning) of your veneers, avoid hard chewing and biting forces on them, and have a dentist-made nightguard which you wear "forever" to protect your veneers. Veneers are designed and made for your bite, your needs, your esthetic goals, and your particular tooth situation.

They may be made of different types of porcelain, depending on your esthetic and strength needs. They are bonded to the teeth, structurally as shown in the diagram.

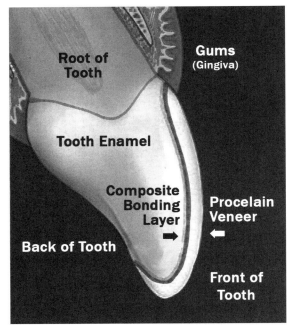

Veneers:

The procedure by the dentist, with the patient

1. Evaluate the smile you have: tooth shape, size, color, length, alignment, lip support, esthetics, phonetics, structural integrity, spacing, and bite.

2. Determine the smile you want, including all the factors above.

3. Make impressions, models of the teeth, jaw relations of how the teeth bite and function together. Take photographs, x-rays, etc.

4. Design the smile in wax on the models.

5. Make matrices of the smile "wax-up" to transfer the designed smile to the mouth.

6. Make a "trial smile" on the teeth, in the mouth, using the matrices from the lab wax-up to form tooth material in the mouth in the look and shape of the proposed veneers.

7. Make changes as desired for esthetics, phonetics, function, etc.

8. Capture the desired changes in a new impression.

9. Prepare the teeth and make impressions (impressions: traditional or digital)

10. Perform provisionalization to protect the teeth (temporary veneers while the final ones are fabricated).

11. Make the veneers in the desired shape, size, etc. using the previous impressions and matrices as guides. The porcelain veneers may be stacked porcelain (more subtle esthetics), "pressed" porcelain (stronger with less subtle esthetics), "milled" porcelain (CAD-CAM; strong) or a combination of the three, to form the final veneers.

12. Seat, bond, and finish the veneers – including many intricate, detailed steps; must be done meticulously.

13. Finish and refine the veneers, bonding material, and the bite.

14. Fabricate a nightguard for long-term protection, and use meticulous home care with brushing, flossing, fluorides, and avoidance of excessive forces on your veneers.

By the time your veneers are completed, we will have designed them at least four times: in our mind, on the models (in wax), on the teeth, (in provisional materials), and again on the teeth (in porcelain, bonded).

With proper forethought, planning, design, and treatment execution, porcelain veneers can truly give you that smile you have always wanted!

"Coming from a person who loves to smile, my teeth are very, very important. I've always had dental work (bonding) performed on my front teeth, but the effects were not long lasting.

After a visit with Dr. Finkel, he informed me about the difference in bonding and veneers. I was concerned about the process, but Dr. Finkel's attention to detail and his well-trained staff helped to alleviate many of my concerns.

Once my porcelain veneers were placed on top of my teeth as a trial, I fell in love! Obviously "Doc" loved them too, because he started to hum one of his tunes. He does a GREAT JOB!

I have received so many compliments on my teeth that I'm beginning to share the benefits of bleaching and veneers with everyone! This has been an amazing time for me. My confidence has sky-rocketed so much that Doc's staff even calls me "Ms. Hollywood."

Chonda

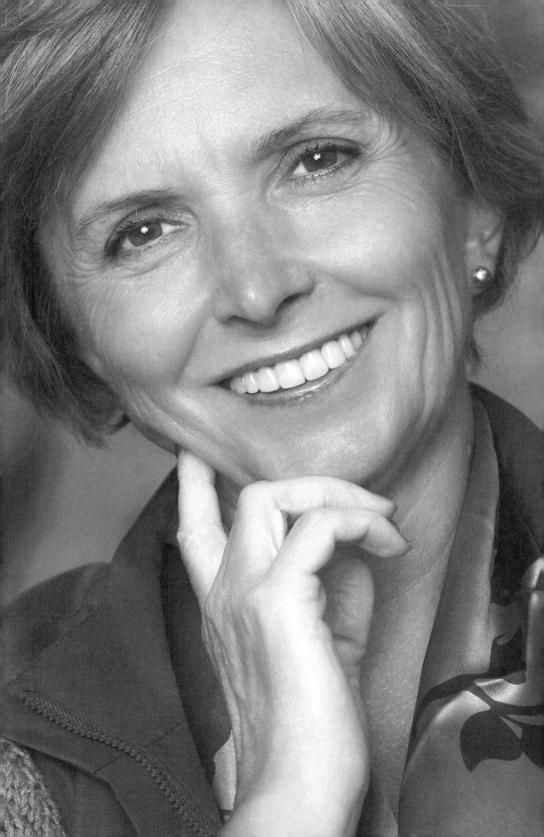

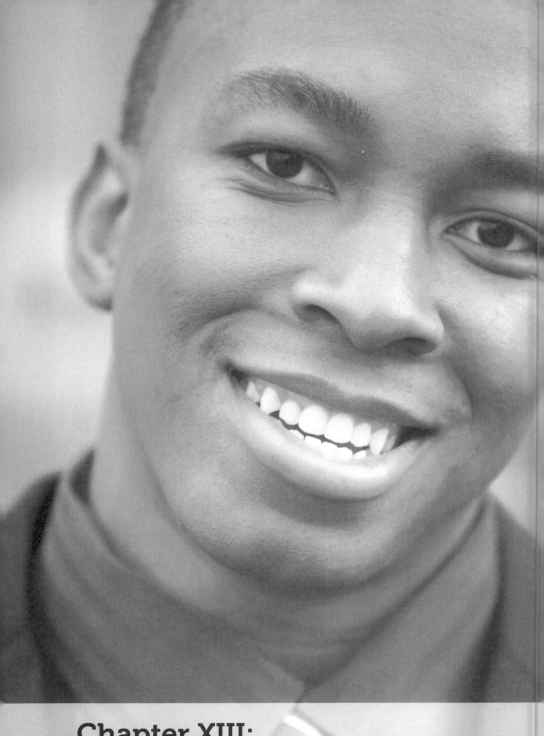

Chapter XIII:
Crowns

Crowns

Crowns (or "caps") are dental restorations which cover the top of a tooth to replace decayed, broken, or missing parts of the tooth and make it whole.

Crowns fit over your tooth like a thimble over the tip of your finger to strengthen the remaining tooth, restore your ability to chew, or to act as retainers (abutments) for a fixed partial denture tooth replacement (or "bridge"). Crowns are also made to fit on implants to create a tooth where there was a gap from a missing tooth.

There are many types of crowns; many margin (design) types and many different crown materials. The type of crown chosen is usually based on tooth position, color, condition, and location; maximizing form, function, durability, and esthetics.

Types of Crowns

1. **Full Gold (yellow or white gold) Crown:** A shell of yellow or white gold fitting over a tooth, replacing lost tooth structure, restoring full shape, strength, and bite to the tooth. This is the strongest, most durable crown available and the best choice for a high-stress tooth for which you want to minimize future treatment needs.

2. **Onlay or Partial Gold Crown:** All biting points ("cusps") of the tooth are covered and strengthened by the gold shell, allowing us to save much of the sides of the tooth. This type of crown combines strength, durability, and conservation of tooth structure.

3. **Porcelain fused to Metal Crown:** A metal casting (shell) with porcelain fused over and around it; this has strength, longevity, and looks like a tooth. It has served dental patients well for years and is

cemented to place; it may show some metal, especially on the inside and near the gums. While not quite as esthetic as all-porcelain crowns, its strength and seal at the edges makes it a good choice for crowns on back teeth, especially molars where esthetics are still a concern. More tooth removal is required for a porcelain-to-metal crown, so it is not quite as conservative as a gold crown. The porcelain is harder than tooth enamel; it can break at seating or in the future. Also, the hardness can create problems if used on second molar teeth due to the increased biting trauma over the years; it does not "wear in" and adapt as do natural teeth or gold crowns.

4. **All-Ceramic (Cemented) Crowns:** These crowns are made totally of ceramic/porcelain; usually of a dense, opaque, inner core of high strength ceramic (zirconia) with overlying esthetic porcelain fused on. While highly esthetic, there are still some compromises with exact fit and with chipping of the overlying porcelain; improvements need to continue. The dense, hard, inner core is strong but can be difficult to work through if the tooth needs future therapy, such as a root canal.

The all-Zirconia crowns, while super-strong, still have some minor problems with fit, are so hard that they can be difficult to adjust, and can later cause bite problems with other teeth.

These all-Zirconia and partial-Zircona crowns are fabricated utilizing CAD-CAM (Computer-Aided-Design....Computer-Aided-Manufacture) milling technology and are taking over a larger share of the dental crown marketplace as they are much less labor-intensive and use no (costly) metal. As a result, they are less expensive to fabricate for the dental laboratory, the dentist, and patient. These will improve in fit and use as time goes on.

5. **All-Porcelain (Bonded) Crowns:** These crowns are fabricated using either CAD-CAM technology ("milled") or lost-wax technology ("pressed"). CAD-CAM or milling technology involves making a digital/virtual impression of the prepared tooth, adjacent teeth, and opposing (biting) teeth and then designing the fit, shape, and bite of the new tooth in virtual (computer) space. A very accurate milling machine carves the tooth (crown) out of a block of the desired material with the desired fit, shape, and bite. The crown is treated (often baked), polished, finished, and ready to seat.

A "pressed" crown is waxed-up (wax-formed) on a physical die (model) of the prepared tooth, surrounded by a hard stone mold of investment material ("invested"), and then the wax is burned out, leaving a tooth-shaped hollow in the mold. The ceramic material is then pressure-forced into the mold in the exact shape of the wax-form tooth. Once baked in the mold, the ceramic is fused and hardened into the crown. It is finished and often receives outer layering of ceramic material for its final shape, bite, and esthetics.

Some of these crowns can be cemented onto the tooth with traditional dental cements; others are bonded to the tooth with newer dental bonding materials to increase their strength and longevity.

These all-ceramic bond-able crowns are the most highly esthetic, but not the most durable, as are full-gold crowns and onlays. They also have the advantage, in the right circumstances, of allowing partial preparation of the tooth, keeping intact more of the natural tooth structure.

Impressions: Traditional or Digital?

Dentistry, for many years, has taken impressions for dental appliances, dentures, crowns, bridges, restorations, etc. with various impression materials in metal and plastic trays over the teeth, in the mouth. These material impressions are highly accurate, and dental models are formed by carefully filling ("pouring up") the impressions with dental stone which then hardens to form the dental model. This dental model is then used to make the dental restoration appliance or crown.

Digital impressions are opening a whole new world of dentistry. A wand, digital scanning device, or special digital camera, using a specific-wavelength-visible light or a laser light, is moved over the teeth to capture a continuous moving video image of the teeth or multiple fixed digital images of the teeth, which the computer can verify and combine into a single digital image. This internal, virtual, image of the teeth is then used to:

a. Create a physical model of the teeth by milling (grinding) it out of plastic, or

b. Create a physical model of the teeth by computer processing (SLA: stereo lithography), or

c. Maintain a digital image of the teeth.

The physical models of the teeth, (a or b) are used by the lab technician to make the dental appliances or restorations. The digital image (c) is used to move directly into digital CAD-CAM manufacture of the appliances or restoration with no intermediate physical model.

The new digital impression technologies are evolving rapidly and quickly improving. Under the pressures of patient comfort, efficiency of time, and ease of dental manufacturing; they will soon be our major technique for dental impressions.

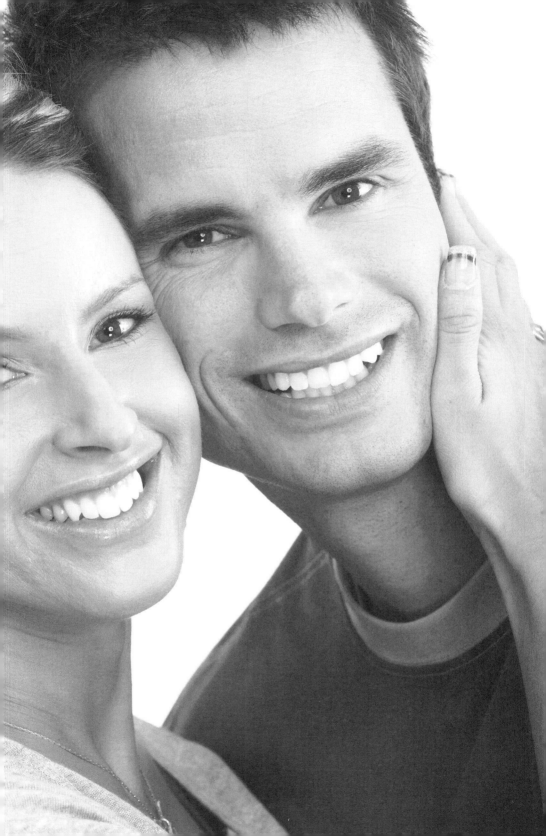

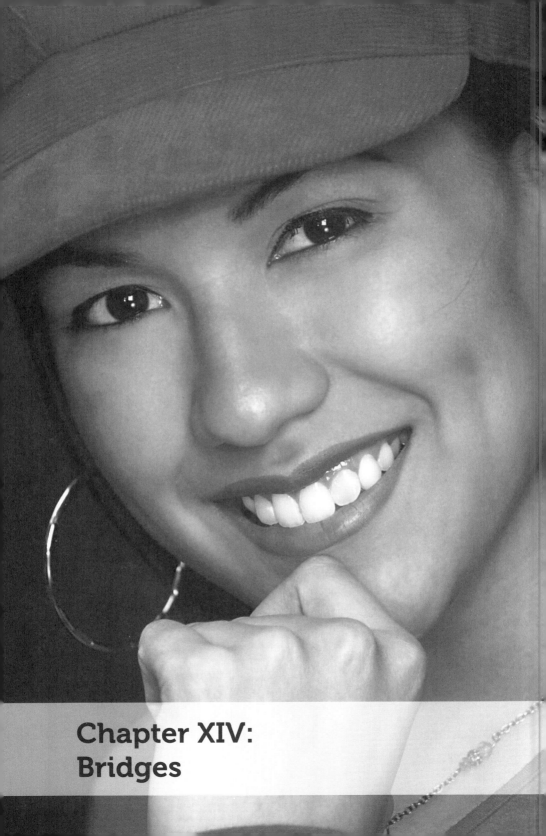

Chapter XIV:
Bridges

Bridges

A dental bridge or "fixed partial denture" is a dental restoration replacing one or more teeth, anchored by crowns or partial crowns to teeth at either end. The missing tooth (pontic) or teeth (pontics) are part of a structure attached to the end teeth (abutments).

Bridges connect one end tooth to another; they can also connect implants together so each implant supports a tooth and one or more false teeth between them.

Bridges can be short (eg. three teeth) or longer, or all around the upper or lower arch. They are tooth supported or implant-supported but not both. Teeth are suspended by fibers (the "periodontal ligament") in the bone and can move and compress before contacting and compressing the bone. Implants are fused to the bone and have much less movement. A bridge attached to teeth and implants will generally loosen from one or the other and will fail.

Bridges can be made for front or back teeth with any and all of the materials and techniques listed for crowns. The more esthetic all-ceramic materials are usually reserved for front teeth, while the stronger materials are used on the back teeth. Materials for bridges must be stronger than those used for individual crowns, and materials for front bridges must emphasize esthetics while those for back teeth must emphasize strength and durability.

When a tooth is missing, a dental bridge is a reasonable replacement for the missing tooth if the adjacent teeth, which will become the end-teeth (abutments) for the bridge, are weak or already heavily-repaired. Crowns would enhance their strength and or appearance. In this case, the crowns are already indicated on these end teeth, so you are treating the damaged teeth and the missing tooth at the same time, with little additional cost for replacing the missing tooth.

When possible, an implant with crown would result in a better force distribution on the teeth and likely last longer than a bridge, but both bone and finances must be available for an implant to be feasible.

When the teeth adjacent to the gap (missing tooth) are healthy, not heavily restored, and in no need of crowns; then an implant with crown, though more costly, is generally more conservative, stronger, and more long-lasting than a bridge. If you are missing a tooth and the adjacent teeth are healthy, then implant restorative dentistry avoids turning a one-tooth problem into a three-tooth problem.

We always strive for health and longevity in our dentistry, so please discuss with us which replacement option, bridge or implant, is right for you.

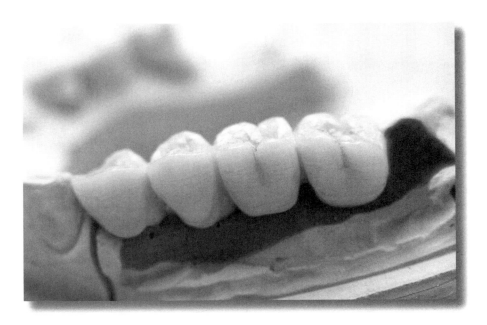

"I have been with Dr. Finkel for over 10 years now, and I cannot see myself going to another dentist.

"I am always greeted by Fran's smiling face, which always sets such a positive tone for my visit.

"Kathy, my hygienist, is so wonderful as well. What I like is she always explains what is going on when others did not. She is very thorough but very gentle when probing and/or flossing.

"As for Dr. Finkel, he too was always smiling and it never makes me feel like my teeth are not important to him. He explains things that he is watching, and areas I need to pay more attention to so as to prevent issues in the future.

"When I check out, both Fran and Tammy are there to help me with all the confusion that dental insurance can bring. They always clarify things for me which is very helpful and comforting knowing they are always watching out for me.

"Again, Dr. Finkel and his team are fun, professional, and very supportive. I've never been to a better dentistry team."

Steve

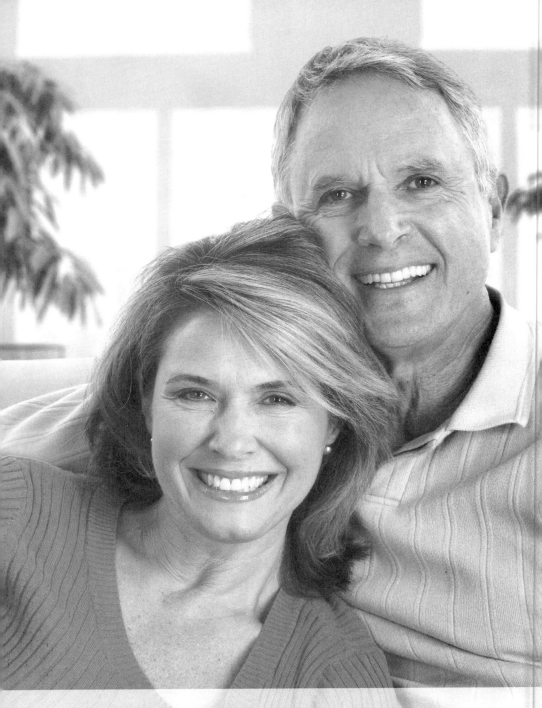

Chapter XV:
Dentures and Partial Dentures

Dentures and Partial Dentures

Dentures (full dentures, complete dentures) are acrylic replacements for all the teeth in the upper or lower arch of the jaws. Partial dentures replace some (not all) of the teeth in the upper or lower arch and hook on the remaining teeth or rest on the remaining teeth and gums. Partial dentures are also known as "removable partial dentures."

Many people think of dentures as a cheap replacement for teeth and an inevitable side effect of growing old. We do know that most people, with proper dental care, can keep their teeth for a lifetime, but many people reach the stage of poor dental health where that is no longer possible. For some, dentures or partial dentures are the most cost-effective and time-effective way of regaining their smile. It is important to know that not all dentures are created equal. While some are made properly, functionally, and well, others are made cheaply, quickly, and poorly and are very unsatisfactory.

Well-made dentures, while not a replacement for your natural teeth, are often quite successful at revitalizing your smile, function, and confidence. Dentures are not part of your body; they are not locked into your gums. They sit on top of your gums. Some dentures and partial dentures look pretty good; many don't. Because dentures sit on top of your gums, the force of chewing goes through the dentures to the soft tissue and bone underneath. Frequently, the soft tissue under a full or partial denture develops painful sore spots. The compression of the bone caused by the chewing on dentures inevitably, over time, leads to loss of bone.

The loss of bone occurs in both height and width. Bone loss of the upper and lower jaws, over time, leads to wrinkles and, for many, facial disfigurement. Bone loss itself makes dentures more difficult to wear and, over time, there is just less bone to rest on. As we age, it becomes harder to wear dentures as a result of loss of bone support and thinning of the tissue over the bone.

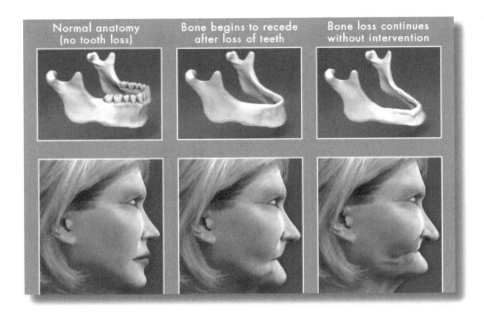

As we age, our capacity for accommodation decreases. We see that on all sorts of levels. We see it in our athletic ability and in our stamina. It should not be a shock or surprise that our ability to accommodate dentures decreases as we grow older.

Many dentures are made poorly (cheaply) for economic reasons. Patients are not aware of the options. If dentures are not custom-made to fit your face, personality, and chewing mechanism; you may quickly develop that "denture look." Worse, a poorly fitting denture accelerates bone loss which worsens the fit which further worsens the bone loss. This continues in a dwindling spiral with the denture wearer suffering the most. Also, dementia appears to be aggravated by a bad bite (especially with bad dentures) and the resultant improper brain function.

We also know that the average denture wearer should have their dentures relined or remade within one year of receiving them. After three years, another reline is probably necessary. After seven years, a new set is needed. Unfortunately, few denture wearers adhere to this schedule of care. In fact, the average denture wearer goes to a dentist only once every 14.9 years! There is a huge gap between what should be and what the public typically does. This failure to see a need for care and receive it, makes the denture experience worse and puts the denture wearer at risk for increased oral cancer, especially for smokers.

Quality Dentures
What is a quality denture and how is it different from a cheap one?

Cheap dentures are made with quick impressions, inaccurate bite techniques, poor materials, and little time. They may serve as "teeth," but rarely do they fit comfortably, function well, look good, or inspire confidence. Their greatest attribute is "cheap"; that is, low cost. Many denture "mills" specialize in cheap, quick, dentures; many of these dentures do not work well and stay in the glass or in the drawer, used only as "social teeth" or "party teeth."

A quality denture is not cheap or quickly made. It is a functional "prosthesis" that helps you enjoy comfort, dining, socializing, and self-confidence.

Quality dentures start with careful, exact, accurate, impressions. The impressions may be two-stage impressions with a "primary" (first) impression to make a special "custom" impression tray and a more exact "final" (second) impression. They may be detailed, carefully developed primary impressions to capture the details of your oral tissues. From this impression is made an exact model of your gums, remaining teeth, and adjacent oral tissues (cheeks, etc).

When making upper and lower dentures, we use these models to fabricate baseplates (forms that fit the models) and wax rims where the gums and teeth will be placed. The wax rims are then carefully adjusted and modified to establish:

1. Length and level of the upper incisors (front teeth)
2. Level (horizontal plane) of all the upper teeth
3. Proper support of the lips and cheeks
4. Facial midline (center line)
5. Correct jaw position to give the lower facial third proper support
6. Proper esthetics (looks), phonetics (speech), and function (chewing)
7. Proper bite of the upper and lower teeth

Denture teeth are then chosen to match your facial shape, size, and profile. You and your dentist then choose your preferred shade (color). You should be deeply involved in the development of your dentures, and you should provide input into the size, color, bite, position, and function of your teeth.

Your chosen teeth should now be set into the wax rims in the proper position to make your dentures look, function, fit, and sound as you like. The denture "wax-up" is then verified by the dentist and patient, and modified as necessary. Once completely acceptable, this wax-up is processed into acrylic, using the highest quality materials and most accurate techniques, giving you your custom dentures. They are then smoothed, polished, and finished, ready for delivery to you.

Once delivered, the dentures should be adjusted to make them fit and work correctly. All the above steps should be completed with loving care and attention to detail; anything less, or skipping any of the above steps, reflects below-par service and is less than you deserve.

What is an Immediate Denture?

An immediate denture is one that is fabricated while the patient still has his or her teeth and is delivered to the patient the same day the remaining teeth are removed. An immediate denture involves the same steps as above to impress and fabricate the denture(s) while the teeth are still present. The dentures are made to the shape that we calculate the gums will have once the teeth are removed, and the dentures are delivered the same day the teeth are removed, sometimes with reshaping of excess bone, gum, or impinging tissue for improved fit. With an immediate denture, you do not have to be without teeth for even a day!

Immediate dentures do come with some cautions:

1. The new dentures can not be "tried in" to verify esthetics, phonetics (speech), and function prior to tooth extractions and delivery. The new teeth may not fit, function, or look exactly as you wished, but they can usually be modified (at little or no cost), partially re-set (at moderate cost), or totally remade (at greater cost).

2. The gums under the dentures will shrink and change shape after the extractions, and the dentures do not change shape; so the fit will become progressively looser over time.

Relines (adding acrylic inside the denture to accommodate the new shape of the gums) can be done chairside (quicker) or lab-processed overnight (more durable) after the gums heal and change shape. For immediate dentures, you should expect to have relines completed at approximately six months after delivery and 18 months (12 months later) after delivery. Each reline is a separate procedure, at additional cost, not included in the original denture fee.

What should I do if my Dentures need more support?

If your denture is loose or unstable, the first option is a reline to re-establish proper fit. If you still desire greater denture stability or want a denture more fully fixed in place, then mini-implants can be placed into the jaw under the denture, and the denture modified to clasp the mini-implants for stability.

We have great success placing two, four, or more standard implants under a denture to create an implant-retained denture (with 2 implants) or implant-supported denture (with 4 implants). Various attachments and denture modifications are then employed to utilize (attach to) the implants. Sometimes the denture needs to be remade.

Denture adhesives

Denture adhesives have been around a long time. These are used to help stabilize dentures. In the U.S. alone, over 200 million dollars a year is spent buying this material. Evidently a lot of people want removable teeth that don't move around!

However, there is a problem. The greatest use of these glops, globs, powders, and gels is to stabilize dentures that should have been re-made because of bone loss. Besides the taste, these adhesives leave a mess in one's mouth.

The poorer the fit of the dentures, the greater the use of the goop to hold them in place. The poorer the fit, the greater the bone loss caused by the ill-fitting dentures! The very thing that is supposed to be helping is causing more loss of bone!

Is there ever a good use for a denture adhesive? Yes, there is. When a person wants the extra security that the adhesive gives them in public places, an adhesive can help out. No one wants to see a person's teeth fall out onto the plate in a restaurant. The real question is how much should be used? Just a light dusting of powder adhesive should be spread out over the whole denture. That is all that it should take to ratchet up the adherence to the tissues. It is so little that it is barely visible.

If the denture wearer is requiring more than just a little adhesive, then the likelihood is that the dentures should be relined or replaced with better fitting ones.

What about Partial Dentures? ("Partials")

Remember that partial dentures replace some (not all) of the teeth in the upper or lower arch and rest on the remaining teeth and gums. They may have hooks and rest bars to hook 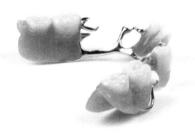 onto the remaining teeth. Given the choice between having no teeth and wearing a full denture, or having some teeth and a partial denture, the partial denture can be a better choice. Why? Because a well-made partial denture distributes the bite forces onto the remaining teeth as much as possible, away from the bone. This requires the partial denture to be rigid, usually made of metal and specifically made to use the teeth as anchors for retention of the partial denture.

Just as with the full denture, the gum and bone underneath the partial denture collapse. In time, the loss of gum and bone can be huge. Partial dentures must be carefully planned and delivered so that the patient can function with them and bone is preserved as much as possible. The goal of a partial is to stabilize tooth positions and to provide chewing surfaces to chew against. It is not as good as chewing on healthy natural teeth.

Here is a real surprise; 40% of partial dentures stay in drawers, worn not at all or just for special occasions. Frequently, a person can chew better without using a partial denture which is poorly made!

Like a full denture, if you must choose a partial denture, get one customized by a real expert to fit very well. It should distribute bite force over as large an area as possible to decrease force on bone. This also means it very well may need far more time effort and expertise to get one well-made. The goal of a well-made partial is to provide chewing surfaces, stabilize the remaining teeth's positions and minimize compressive force onto the bone. Remember that force on bone causes it to melt away over time.

Creating a well-made partial denture is a tall order. Even when done well, many people find partials uncomfortable to wear. Many people consider the hooks of the partial denture fitting onto the remaining teeth to be so unsightly that they refuse to wear them.

Statistically speaking, teeth that anchor partial dentures are more likely to decay or get loose from the force put against them by the partial. If you are saying to yourself, "Why would anyone want a partial denture?", I understand. They should be avoided if possible; it is best to keep your real teeth, have fixed bridges where necessary, and implants where possible.

Some notes on Dentures:

<u>Clicking dentures</u> are usually caused by looseness and poor fit; the dentures may need to be relined or remade.

<u>A denture should be as large as possible</u> and still "go to place" in the mouth. The larger the denture, the greater area over which to distribute chewing force ("the snow-shoe effect") and the less force on the bone and delicate oral tissues.

The size of the denture is limited by the position of the cheeks, lips, tongue, oral floor, and associated muscles (especially the lower). It is always a balance in size between over-all support, muscle position, tongue position, and movement of the cheeks, lips and tongue.

Denture biting force is usually about one eighth the biting force of natural teeth and becomes much less over time.

Final Denture Recommendations

- If you must have dentures, get the best ones possible from an experienced dentist who makes high quality dentures on a regular basis. The dentist should make customized impressions, bite registrations and customized tooth arrangement. Often custom coloring of denture bases is needed to match the color of your gums.

- If you must have dentures, get overdentures (over implants) if you can. These preserve bone better and protect your facial contours better than full dentures.

- Replace your dentures every seven-eight years.

- Get relines every two-four years as needed to keep your dentures fitting and functioning as well as possible.

- Let your mouth rest at least eight hours a day by removing your dentures, usually overnight.

- If it is possible for you, get dental implants to avoid becoming toothless. If you are already a denture wearer, find a way to get dental implants. They can change your life.

Any time that you can use dental implants or natural teeth in a healthy mouth, instead of removable teeth, you are better off.

For some people, dentures are the only solution. In that case, get them made as well as you possibly can. But if possible, choose the alternative, dental implants.

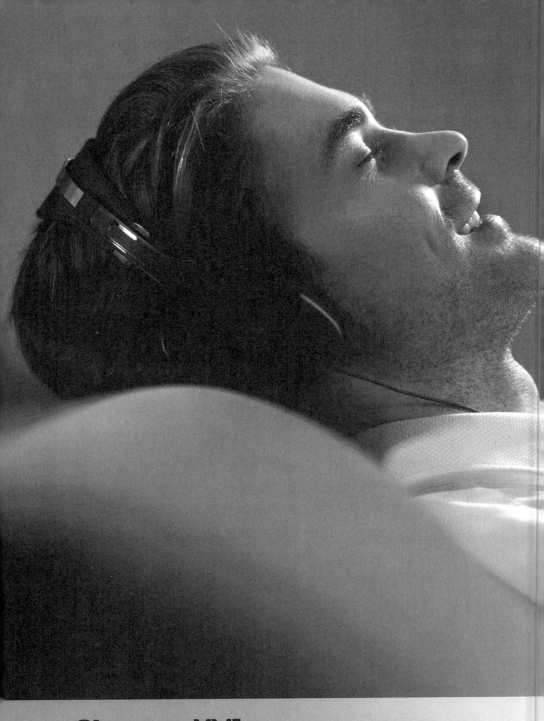

Chapter XVI:
Sedation Dentistry

Sedation Dentistry

Many of our patients would like to be totally relaxed for their dentistry with little or no memory of what was done during their appointment. Some patients have had bad dental experiences earlier in life and some patients have had other distressing medical or life experiences with bad memories easily re-stimulated in the dental chair. For some, being in the dental operatory can re-activate the memories of past surgical procedures or traumas where pain, unconsciousness, and loss of control were present.

Some anxious individuals and some high-energy, very active, individuals simply do not like to stop and slow down. Possibly, they are always thinking of what they "ought" to be doing, and their mind never goes into "relax" mode.

For any of these folks, previously-traumatized, fearful, anxious, or simply high-energy and not easily relaxed, we have some techniques to help them relax for their dentistry, with little or no recollection of their dental treatment.

"Laughing Gas", or Nitrous Oxide

Nitrous Oxide is a gas already present in our air. When used in higher concentration, for medical procedures, it can help us relax during treatment. Medical and dental use of nitrous oxide, highly purified and with proper equipment, is safe and effective. Modern dental oxygen/nitrous-oxide regulators (dispensing equipment) are designed so the patient always receives more oxygen than is present in normal room air; the safety features are a basic part of our equipment so patient well-being is paramount.

Nitrous oxide has been used in dentistry for many years, safely and effectively, to reduce patient anxiety and ease dental treatment. Properly administered, with attention paid to silence and avoiding implanted suggestions, it can be a boon to dental patients. It can lessen anxiety, increase relaxation, and make your dental visit much more enjoyable. The best dental visit is always a gentle one; for those who are anxious and for more involved dental appointments, "laughing gas" can ease your way.

Silence is Golden

During the use of laughing gas, as with deeper sedation and general anesthesia, care must be taken to avoid giving the patient implanted suggestions easily reactivated later in life. During times of lessened consciousness like being drunk, sedated, or under general anesthesia; the individual is still aware of his or her surroundings and can hear and sense what is going on. At these times the analytical part of the mind that filters and analyzes data is "suspended," and the unconscious mind accepts all data as if it is real, valid, and directed at the individual.

At these times, the unconscious mind will pick up data and suggestions as if one is hypnotized and will translate many phrases and instructions into post-hypnotic commands which, unremembered, are taken as rules for later in life. Especially if these periods of lessened consciousness are combined with anxiety, fear or painful experiences, any suggestions picked up can cause us to unknowingly act to follow these "implanted" suggestions/commands when later situations in life bring up similar sensations, memories, or experiences.

During the use of nitrous oxide or deeper sedation, the patient should be protected from hearing phrases that can later by taken as post-hypnotic commands such as "stay still," "don't move," "be quiet," and "stay open wide." Phrases such as "you will hurt a bit," "you won't feel a thing," "you should relax," and "don't think about it," can also be "implanted" in the subconscious as commands one must live by.

Often, the patient, with eyes closed, will be so open to suggestion that instructions from the dentist to staff such as "hold still," "stay right there," or "move faster" can internalized by the patient and unconsciously applied later as hidden commands. Comments such as "things are not going right," "this will hurt later," "you shouldn't do that," and "things just aren't right" may be internalized and later acted out unconsciously without the patient's awareness that he or she is unknowingly acting out a hidden, implanted, command.

During the suggestibility of sedation and lessened consciousness, even statements such as "you will do great," "nothing can go wrong," and "you won't feel a thing" can be instilled in the subconscious mind as a false sense of wellness or invulnerability. Future disregard for normal caution can lead one to errors in judgment if this hidden command is "obeyed."

When a patient is sedated, they are more highly suggestible, so that any instruction can be taken as a post-hypnotic suggestion. Negative ideas can come back as a later depressed, or depressive state; positive commands can come back as a later overly care-free or manic state.

The Golden Rules of Sedation

The two rules for sedation should be:

1. Silence: Anything said during a period of sedation can be later misinterpreted by the patient's unconscious mind.

2. The patient should be informed prior to and after the procedure that anything possibly taken as a post-hypnotic suggestion should be disregarded or "cancelled out."

Conscious Dental Sedation

For some dental patients, an even deeper level of relaxation is necessary for them to receive dental care. Memories of past experiences, anxiety, or fear can cause patients to avoid dental care, and often these folks end up needing even more dentistry. High-energy individuals may not easily "slow down" for their dental appointments.

For these individuals, sedation dentistry can be a blessing. We often combine night-before relaxation medication and sedation medication combined with nitrous oxide for the dental procedure. To help our patients be relaxed for the dental appointment and have little or no memory of what was done, different sedation protocols will be indicated, based on patient anxiety level, patient preference, health status, and length of procedure.

Not to be taken lightly, dental sedation should involve proper patient screening and medical evaluation. Health status, present medications, and potential drug interactions should be reviewed. Proper monitoring of cardiac function, pulse, blood pressure, and blood oxygen levels should occur during sedation and treatment; and your dental team should be properly trained. The previously mentioned adherence to silence and avoidance of mental "implants" should be observed, and proper follow-up instructions should be provided.

Used properly and as indicated, dental conscious sedation is safe and effective in making your dental experience easier and more pleasant.

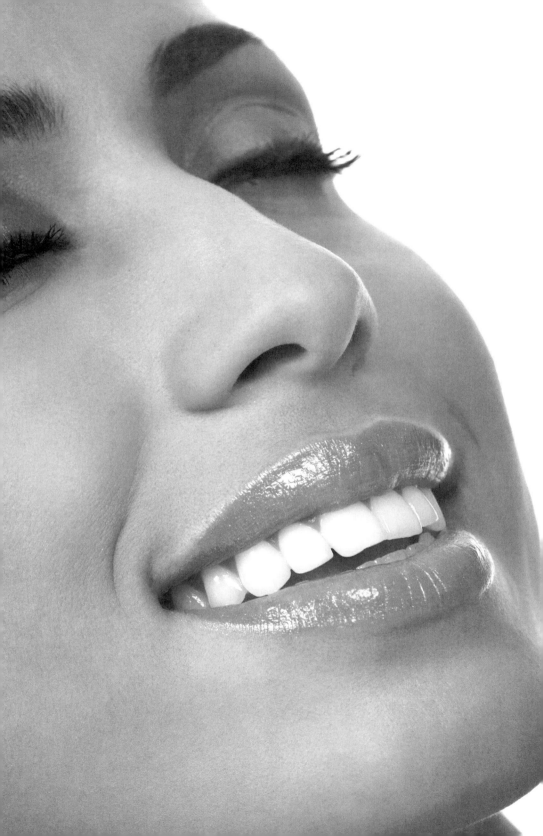

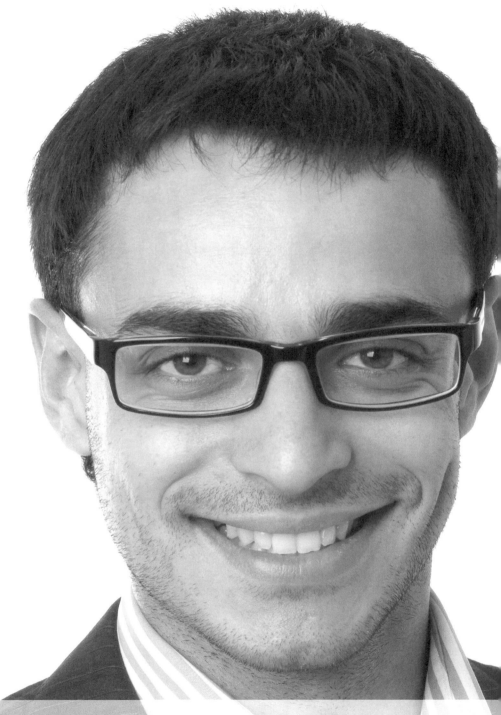

Chapter XVII:
Technology in Dentistry

Some Newer Techniques

Composite (Bonded tooth-colored fillings)

The older silver fillings were once the best we could offer and, in some situations, may still provide the best service. Cavities on molar roots are often best filled with silver amalgam. Resealing cavities at the edges (margins) of crowns may sometimes best be performed with silver amalgam if resources are not available to redo the crown or if the crown is part of an expensive-to-redo bridge. We do very few silver fillings these days, as we prefer to offer our patients the bonding strength, seal and esthetics of bonded tooth-colored composites. Each material has certain advantages and drawbacks; silver amalgam is sometimes more decay-resistant, easier, faster, and cheaper for the patient. Composite bonded fillings, properly done, are more technique-sensitive, time-consuming, and costly to place. The choice is, and always should be, yours.

CAD-CAM: Computer-Aided-Design / Computer-Aided-Manufacture

"Crowns-in-an-hour" or "crowns-in-a-morning" are now being offered by some dental offices, and some dentists have based their dental career on the concept. In dentistry for over two decades, this technique takes a visual digital scan of teeth prepared for crowns, fillings, or bridges. Using visual scans, laser imaging or repeated video scans, a computer builds up a "virtual" image and model of the tooth or teeth to be restored.

The dentist then designs the restoration (crown, inlay, bridge) on the computer model and determines shape, fit, bite (occlusion), and tooth contacts; often using scanned computer models of the adjacent teeth, images of the opposing (biting) teeth, computerized bite scans, and scans of the tooth/teeth prior to preparation. He or she may also access computer-library models of ideal teeth to merge into the computer design. The dentist then instructs the computer to micro-precision mill (grind) the restoration out of the specified material and processes the milled restoration to the final state. The restoration is then bonded or cemented to the tooth without need for a second visit or numbing. Systems such as "CEREC" or "E4D" are in use and have long-term track records. These restorations can last a long time but are more prone to fracture, failure, and early breakdown than "conventional" crowns, and replacement then requires more cost and tooth loss for the patient. Some dentists see this technique as a road to higher profit, as they can complete a crown in one visit (less time) without the cost of the second visit. Many patients see the possible conservative tooth preparation and convenience as well worth the cost and somewhat shortened life-span of the restoration. Some dentists with proper training, skill, and standards can produce truly beautiful and long-lasting restorations with CAD-CAM; others have higher failure rates. This is an area of dentistry truly deserving of frank discussion with your dentist and evaluation of your dental values, including conservation of tooth structure, convenience, and longevity.

Digital dental impressions

The same scanning techniques employed in CAD-CAM dental treatment (above) may be employed to create a digital impression and physical model of teeth prepared for restoration without use of impression trays and impression material. Many patients would appreciate not having to wait while impression material sets up in their mouth, and many dentists would appreciate the ability to immediately visualize areas of the tooth preparation which could be modified or refined for a better end-result.

There are still "bugs" to be worked out of these systems as dental laboratories and dentists are finding variable results with the different available systems. As of now, 2012, these systems need to be improved and calibrated for accuracy, but digital impression techniques are likely the wave of the future and will probably slowly phase out real-material dental impressions for much of dentistry. Real-material dental impressions are currently our standard for reliability and accuracy and will likely remain so for larger dental impressions used in larger cases, dentures, and specialized dental situations.

"Laser Bleaching:" one-hour bleaching

These techniques are great marketing tools and wonderful for quick-start bleaching when a patient needs immediate results. However, university studies show that bleaching occurs because of the chemicals used on the teeth, not the laser- or light-activation. After one week, the results of in-office, one-hour, "laser" bleaching are the same with or without use of the light and within a week, both revert to near-baseline (original tooth color) shade results. The in-office bleaching does more for the dentist than the patient, is more costly, causes more sensitivity, and decreases the micro-hardness of the tooth enamel. (Long-term effects, if any, of this decrease in enamel micro-hardness have not been clarified or quantified)

Regular dentist-supervised home bleaching with accurate dental-office-made trays from models of your teeth, has been shown to be safe, predictable, comfortable, less-sensitivity-causing, and capable of long-term, stable, predictable results. If you need immediate bleaching results for a wedding or re-union in two days, then in-office, one-hour bleaching may be worth the additional cost and sensitivity. Otherwise, proper tray bleaching is usually a better value and a better choice for long-term results.

Air-Abrasion tooth preparation for fillings

Air-abrasion, like a miniature sand-blaster, can be used to prepare a tooth for bonding, remove decay, or prepare a cavity for a filling. It is messier than use of a dental drill but can sometimes eliminate the noise of the dental drill and the need for numbing. Tooth preparation is slower and less exact than with a dental drill and it cannot remove old amalgam fillings adequately. This technique is often useful in specialized dental situations and warrants discussion with your dentist.

Cancer detection systems – for oral cancer

Oral cancer screening has traditionally been performed by the dentist and hygienist visually, looking for changes in the appearance of oral tissues and then biopsy (surgical removal and microscopic examination) of tissue as necessary. Unfortunately, oral cancer (usually squamous cell carcinoma) is often highly destructive and often fatal because of poor visual screening and oral cancer's ability to remain visually undetected.

Cancer screening techniques that are in use or in development, and that should be welcomed by the patient are:

A. **Visual Screening:** by the dentist or hygienist with removal and biopsy of suspicious areas of tissue as indicated.

B. **Cytology Smears (Oral CDX):** similar to a Pap Smear, in which a small brush is used to scrape tissue cells from the surface of a suspicious lesion in the mouth. These cells are preserved and scanned, looking for abnormal changes indicative of cancer. Depending on results, these lesions are observed, lightly removed, or more deeply excised.

C. **Specialized Light Scanning Instruments (Velscope):** This instrument shines a special-wavelength filtered light on the oral (mouth) tissues which are visually scanned for dark or abnormal patches when viewed through a special scope. When located, these patches are tested and, if not merely inflamed or blood-filled areas, are suspected of cellular cancer-prone changes and biopsied.

D. **Chemical/Light Screening for Oral Cancers (Visilite System):** In this oral cancer screening system, one rinses with weak acetic acid (diluted vinegar) and then with a blue dye solution (Toluidine Blue). Abnormal cancer-prone tissues pick up the blue dye to a greater degree, indicating cellar changes that may be, or lead to, oral cancer. A special blue-filtered light is also used to scan the mouth for suspicious changes.

E. **Salivary Tests for Cancer-Causing Oral Viruses:** Certain human virus cause wart-like lesions, sometimes visible and sometimes not, that can become cancerous. One salivary test checks for presence of this virus, indicating higher risk for development of oral caner.

F. **Salivary Test for Oral Cancer:** Oral cancer (usually squamous cell carcinoma) produces special protein markers (cellular chemicals) that reveal the presence of oral cancer, even when not visually evident. When the dentist adds a special regent (chemical) to the saliva of a patient who has this oral cancer, a color change occurs, indicating the presence of these protein markers and the presence of oral cancer.

A positive result for E. and F. then requires more detailed examination to locate the suspicious area in the mouth for evaluation and testing. Oral cancer is easily overlooked and easily mis-diagnosed. Early detection and treatment improves outcomes and saves lives.

Other salivary diagnostics

Many tests using only your saliva are currently in development, testing, and marketing for other diseases such as:

1. Genetic susceptibility to periodontal disease

2. Presence of specific periodontal-disease-causing bacteria

3. HIV/AIDS and other viral diseases

4. Diabetes

5. Liver Disease

6. Body organ cancers

7. Whole-body inflammation from chronic infections, which increases the likelihood of stroke, heart disease, diabetes, and a whole host of other problems

8. Many other tests are in development; we look to the future for what else your mouth can tell us about your overall health.

Dental Implants

One of the greatest innovations to occur in dentistry in recent history: Please see our chapter on Implants (p. 112).

Bonded Veneers and Crowns

The ability to bond porcelain shells and porcelain crowns to conservatively-prepped teeth is also one of the greatest changes in dentistry in recent years. Please see our chapters on Bonded Veneers and Crowns (pp. 134 and 142).

Lasers: Boon or Bust?

More recent technologies have a place in dentistry, but the new technology should fill a need and solve a problem; not be a solution waiting for a problem. The technology should improve your dentistry, not be mere dazzle and flash.

Lasers in Dentistry

Lasers are becoming more common in dentistry and can serve many functions in your dental care. A laser (Light Amplification by Stimulated Emission of Radiation) light is a type of light of all one wavelength. An electronic diode, liquid, gas, or crystal is stimulated (activated) to produce a beam of focused, coherent (in-phase) light which can be controlled and used to beam light energy into or onto many materials to create desired effects. Some possibilities in dentistry:

1. **Cavity Detection:**

    Lasers can be shined into a tooth and measured for bounce-back (reflectance) indicating healthy tooth structure versus absorption and re-emission of the laser light (fluorescence) indicating tooth breakdown (cavity). Devices such as the Diagnodent, using these principles, can help detect cavities under the tooth surface before they can be seen by eye.

2. **Curing of Composite Materials:**

    Composite tooth-colored, bonded filling materials can be activated and set (cured) with laser light so your dentist can place and shape (sculpt) the material to fill cavities and reshape teeth and then, when shaping is completed, light-cure the material to set and bond ("cure") it. Lasers can be used for quick, intense cure of the material as can other types of curing lights.

3. **Accelerated Healing:**

    Some studies (mainly European) indicate that low level helium-neon (red) laser light, as used in office pointers, can accelerate wound repair and speed the body's natural healing process after mouth surgery and mouth trauma. Other lasers can stimulate healing of deeper tissues.

    More intense laser therapy can also be used to treat herpes virus lesions ("cold sores") and recurrent apthous ulcers ("RAU" or "canker sores") on the lips, cheeks, and gums.

4. **Removal of Excess Oral Soft Tissue:**

    Laser energy can be used to remove ("ablate") excess gum tissue to recontour the "cuff" of gums around the teeth. This technique allows for access to cavities and tooth areas to be repaired which would normally be hidden under the gum.

    After removal of the in-the-way gum tissue, the dentist has visual and physical access to see and perform needed dental treatment, including access, inside the gums, to implants being restored with crowns.

    Lasers can also be used to reshape the gums around the front teeth so short-looking teeth can be made to look longer, more natural, and more esthetic. This is called "gingival esthetic recontouring" for a healthier-looking smile.

    The laser can also be used to remove, or ablate, benign bumps and growths in the mouth and to reshape the soft part of the gums so you can more effectively clean the teeth with brush and floss. The teeth can then be kept cleaner and more free of the bacteria that cause cavities and gum disease.

An Important Note:

Except for working around implants, all the laser functions of intra-oral (in the mouth) soft-tissue removal and reshaping can be accomplished with another technology: electro-surgery or radio-surgery. This uses a fine wire contact ("electrode") like a scalpel but with high-frequency radio-wave-like energy pulses to carve, shape, and remove layers of tissue. This technique has been with us for many decades, improved over time, and works very effectively and cleanly. While not generally used around metal implants or in patients with cardiac pacemakers, it is a fine technique with good results and nice healing. While not as flashy as the laser, it is a fine technique with a proven record.

5   **Tooth Preparation for Cavities, Inlays, and Crowns:**

Currently, lasers are not often used for full crown preparations on teeth because of the slow nature of laser tooth preparation. They may, however, be used to prepare teeth for fillings by removing cavities (decay) and shaping for the final filling material. The advantage of laser preparation for cavities is elimination of the dental drill noise and sometimes avoiding the need for anesthesia (numbing). In many cases, however, use of a dental handpiece (drill) is necessary for final preparation of the tooth to receive the filling material. Lasers should not be used for removing old silver amalgam fillings.

6.   **Lasers in Root Canal Therapy:**

Lasers may also be used for cleaning, shaping, and sterilization of root canal spaces inside the tooth prior to final root canal filling and sealing (obturation). The laser energy may be focused directly on the inner walls of the tooth and roots or, in a process called "photo-acoustic streaming," used to activate a liquid placed inside the roots.

This high-energy activation with laser energy enables the liquid to clean and sterilize the root canal spaces. The sterilization of the root canal spaces can also be accomplished with vibrating (sonic and ultra-sonic) root canal files in conjunction with special irrigating solutions.

7. **Lasers in Periodontal (gum) Therapy:**

    Lasers can treat deeper gum pockets, sterilizing them to eliminate the disease-causing bacteria. Other instruments are still required to fully clean and prepare the root surface for healing; some studies show this combination of traditional and laser therapy to be beneficial in reducing the periodontal disease pockets and resolving the localized infections. Reshaping of the soft-tissue (gums) part of the pockets is another use for the laser, as is reshaping of the underlying bone and gums so you can be effective with your brush and floss. These techniques serve only to reshape the gum structures for cleansability by the patient; they do not "cure" gum disease. Once begun, gum disease (periodontitis) is managed by proper home care, frequent professional cleanings, and additional therapies as required. Oral medications to slow down bone loss, localized application of medications into the gum pockets, and specialized home care techniques may be added to your periodontal therapy as needed.

    A cautionary note on dental lasers:

    Over-treatment with lasers is possible and this author has seen cases where over-enthusiastic use of the laser therapy to reshape the bone and gums has resulted in loss of teeth and the surrounding bone. Your dentist must have significant training to make your periodontal laser therapy effective and safe.

Some dentists have also claimed amazing results at using laser dental therapy to "regrow" bone previously lost around teeth. To date, these claims are unproven and these results are not supported by published research. Any such claims of the dentist's ability to use lasers to help "regrow" bone around teeth may turn out to be exaggerated and should be viewed with skepticism. Future objective (unbiased) studies are needed to determine how much of laser therapy is:

a) A breakthrough in dental care, or

b) Another effective tool in our dental armamentarium, or

c) A good tool for us but no real improvement in our dental techniques, or

d) Marketing flash to impress patients, or

e) A fancy solution to problems already well-handled by our current techniques.

It seems obvious that lasers in dentistry will be helpful to make certain dental treatments easier, faster, and more comfortable yet not replace similar tools which currently show great benefits and long-term results.

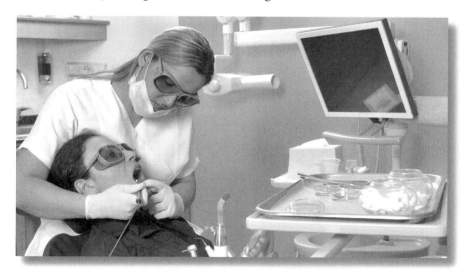

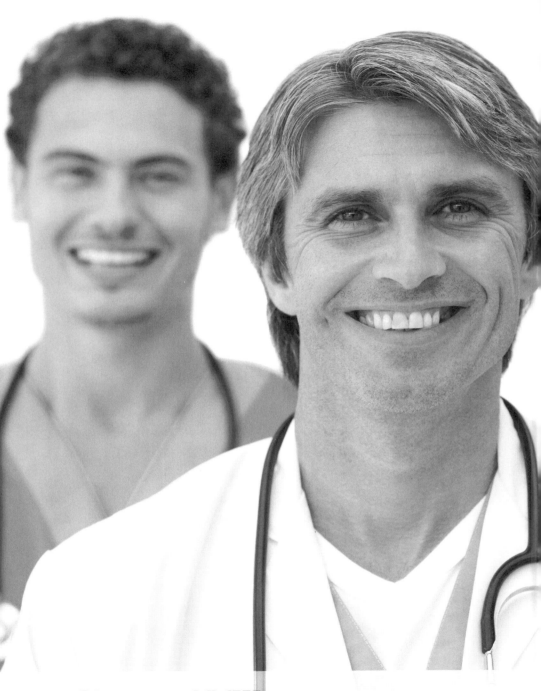

Chapter XVIII:
Dentistry & Medical Problems

Dentistry & Medical Problems

Modern medicine has shown us that there is an intimate relationship between oral health and general health. Infection in the mouth, such as periodontal disease (gum disease), can cause such ills as pre-term labor, low birth weight babies, strokes, heart disease, and kidney disease. Bite problems can cause headaches, facial pain, weakness and fatigue. Sleep problems (which we can treat) may cause tiredness, high blood pressure, and other systemic ailments. An oral infection can also spread to other areas in the head, neck, and face and can affect other organs in the body. Prevention and treatment of dental-related problems is essential to maintaining full body health.

The Mouth - a Mirror of Health

During routine dental examination, we check for more than tooth decay, gum disease, and orthodontic problems. During an oral exam, we're looking for signs of everything from cancer to diabetes to eating disorders.

The mouth is often called the body's "barometer" or "mirror" of health because it's easy to observe and because many health problems and diseases have oral signs or symptoms.

The mouth serves as the body's built-in alarm system. Signs and symptoms orally can indicate trouble elsewhere. More than 40 serious ailments can manifest themselves in the mouth and the tongue, including diabetes, cancer, hepatitis, infection, and Crohn's disease.

As members of the health care team, dentists have been trained to recognize signs of diseases with oral manifestations and to refer patients to physicians for further examination and treatment.

To us, a loose tooth may be a sign of gum disease and bleeding gums the result of overzealous brushing. But each of these symptoms could mean a much more serious illness and the difference between life and death.

We are often the first health care professionals to detect early signs of oral cancer. Warning signals of oral cancer include white, smooth, or scaly patches in the mouth or on the lips; swelling or lumps in the mouth; sores on the lips, gums, and mouth that do not heal, and repeated bleeding in the mouth without apparent cause.

Other disorders that can show up in the mouth include:

- **Vitamin A deficiencies:** A burning or sore tongue is a common symptom of iron, folic acid, and vitamin B12 deficiencies. Bleeding gums can be a warning not only of gum disease but also of a vitamin C deficiency.
- **Diabetes:** Early signs can include red, swollen gums and teeth that are sensitive to tapping, biting, or pressure.
- **Leukemia:** Signs can include sores inside the cheek, in the throat and on the tonsils and lips.
- **Bulimia:** The compulsive pattern of binge eating and then vomiting can lead to a loss of enamel and dentin on the inner (tongue) sides of teeth. Often, this enamel loss is the only outward sign that something is wrong. Thus, dentists are frequently the first to diagnose this eating disorder.
- **Infectious mononucleosis:** Symptoms include inflamed gums and tiny hemorrhage (bleeding) spots on the roof of the mouth.
- **Sinusitis:** The inflammation of the sinus cavity can be mistaken for a toothache.
- **Bleeding Disorders:** Bleeding gums and oral bleeding may indicate clotting problems or genetic disorders.

Dentists can also detect early stages of herpes, AIDS, syphilis, gonorrhea, hypertension, and Multiple Sclerosis from oral symptoms.

Regular dental examinations have always been the best way to maintain healthy teeth and gums. But they help you care for the rest of your body too.

Eating Disorders

Those among us with eating disorders are often unhappy. If your problem is eating too much, we can help with a dental appliance that will slow down your eating until your body's satisfaction with food can catch up with your appetite. Your body has time to enjoy the sensation of eating, digestion, and fullness (which usually lags 20+ minutes behind the actual food) before you have over-eaten. Working with your medical provider, we can help.

If your problem is anoxeria and/or bulimia, we will often find dental (tooth) changes from lack of saliva, acid erosion from regurgitation, acid erosion from acidic drinks (eg. diet sodas), and excessive wear from tooth grinding. In a supportive and non-judgmental atmosphere, we can help you protect your teeth from lack of saliva, the effects of acids, and grinding. We offer support to help you keep your teeth healthy and whole, not criticism, judgment, or invalidation. We want to be part of the answer and a safe part of your support team.

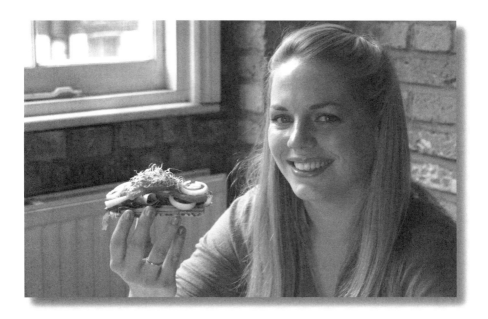

Diabetes & Health

What is periodontal disease?

Periodontal (gum) disease may result from gingivitis, an inflammation of the gums usually caused by the presence of bacteria in plaque. Plaque is the sticky film that accumulates on teeth both above and below the gum line. Without regular dental checkups, periodontal disease may result if gingivitis is left untreated. It also can cause inflammation and destruction of tissues surrounding and supporting teeth, gums (gingiva), bone, and fibers which hold the gums to the teeth.

A number of factors increase the probability of developing periodontal disease, including diabetes, smoking, poor oral hygiene, diet, and genetic makeup; it is the primary cause of tooth loss in adults.

How are periodontal disease and diabetes related?

It is estimated that 26 million people in the U.S., or 8.5% of the population, have diabetes, of which 25% are undiagnosed. Another 80 million people are prediabetic and also at risk.

Studies have shown that diabetics are more susceptible to the development of oral infections and periodontal disease than those who do not have diabetes. Oral infections tend to be more severe in diabetic patients than non-diabetic patients. And, diabetics who do not have good control over their blood sugar levels tend to have more infections and oral health problems. These infections occur more often after puberty and in aging patients.

What types of problems could I experience?

Diabetics may experience diminished salivary flow and burning mouth or tongue. Dry mouth (xerostomia) also may develop, causing an increased incidence of decay. Gum recession has been found to occur more frequently and more extensively in moderately- and poorly-controlled diabetic patients because plaque responds differently, creating more harmful proteins in the gums of diabetics. To prevent problems with bacterial infections in the mouth, your dentist may prescribe antibiotics, medicated mouth rinses, and more frequent cleanings.

How can I stay healthy?

Make certain to take extra good care of your mouth and have dental infections treated immediately. Diabetics who receive good dental care and have good insulin control typically have a better chance at avoiding gum disease and tooth loss.

Diet, oral care, and exercise may be the most important changes that diabetics can make to improve their quality of life and their oral health.

Diabetic patients should be sure their medical and dental care providers are aware of their medical history and periodontal status. To keep teeth and gums strong, diabetic patients should be aware of their blood sugar levels in addition to having their triglycerides and cholesterol levels checked on a regular basis. These may have a direct correlation with your chances of developing periodontal disease.

What is the best time to receive dental care?

If your blood sugar is not under control, talk with both your dentist and physician about receiving elective dental care. Dental procedures should be as short and stress free as possible. Also, make morning appointments because blood glucose tends to be under better control at this time of day.

If you have a scheduled appointment, eat and take your medication as directed. See your dentist on a regular basis, keep him or her informed of your health status, and keep your mouth in good health.

Dentistry and Metabolic Syndrome

What is Metabolic Syndrome and how does it relate to dentistry?

Metabolic Syndrome is a systemic disease syndrome consisting of some combination of:

a. Obesity
b. Diabetes/Insulin resistance
c. Elevated triglycerides
d. Low HDL
e. High blood pressure.

Metabolic Syndrome has been associated with Sleep Disordered Breathing; breathing problems during sleep cause disruption of the normal sleep cycle with resultant increase in the hormones of hunger and decrease in the hormones of satiety/satisfaction. Eating is then increased under the drive of this hormone imbalance and to provide the energy to overcome the fatigue of sleep-deprivation. Weight is then seen to increase, worsening diabetic stressors.

Sleep cycle disruption also increases the death of insulin-producing pancreatic cells, suppresses insulin production in the remaining cells, and results in the development of Type II Diabetes. Ongoing sleep problems increase the severity of the diabetes, make it more difficult to treat, and help initiate the other aspects of Metabolic Syndrome.

The infection and inflammation of Periodontal Disease are also associated with Metabolic Syndrome. Treatment of Periodontal Disease and dental treatment of Sleep Disordered Breathing can aid in the treatment of this syndrome.

Insulin & Cortisol... Double Trouble

Blood Sugar Basics

Want to get leaner? Have more energy? Achieve and sustain optimum health? Insulin is a storage hormone. Excess insulin cancels out all the above benefits. And excess insulin will trigger the release of another problem—excess cortisol.

Protein and fat trigger the release of virtually no insulin whatsoever. This is why you can eat lean protein and/or good fats and oils by themselves. Carbohydrates are what trigger insulin release—either too much carbohydrate at any one time ("carbo-hydrating") or any carbohydrate eaten by itself.

A classic scenario: you wake up in the morning. You experience hunger—which means your blood sugar is low (hypoglycemia). You grab a glass of orange juice and a toaster strudel. By the way, toaster breakfast tarts now outsell the number one selling breakfast cereal, Sugar Frosted Flakes, two to one. They taste sweet and good. But, because they are nearly pure carbohydrates, and highly processed carbs at that, they are broken down into glucose almost instantly and cause your blood sugar level to spike. Your brain—which can only burn glucose—has a fairly narrow range of tolerance. Spiking glucose shocks your pancreas into action. Overreacting, your pancreas secrets a gush of insulin into your blood stream in a valiant effort to stem the drastically rising tide of blood sugar.

Insulin, being a storage hormone, converts the excess glucose into triglycerides (blood fat) and stores this fat in your fat cells. In the process, there is NO fat coming out of your fat cells. It is ALL going in. And with what is known as insulin over-shoot, your blood sugar level dives and you end up in rebound hypoglycemia, a lower blood sugar level than when you started out in the first place.

The Cortisol Kicker

As if this were not bad enough, another powerful hormone is released to bring your blood sugar back up—cortisol. Cortisol is a very potent stress hormone. Prehistorically, it was meant to be released then rapidly burned off. Chronically elevated cortisol causes no end of problems. Hypercortisolism creates a state of inflammation in your body leading to everything from arthritis to heart disease. According to some researchers, cortisol is a major cause of neurological degeneration including memory loss and Alzheimer's disease. Cortisol is "catabolic", meaning it wastes both muscle and bone and is, therefore, a major cause of osteoporosis.

If you've read the best single book on physiology stress, *Why Zebras Don't Get Ulcers*, by the world's authority Stanford Sapolsky Ph.D., you know cortisol is a major stress hormone and is very damaging. If you've read Dr. Barry Sears' most recent book, *Toxic Fat: When Good Fat Turns Bad,* you know that cortisol is a major ageing accelerator. Dr. Barry Sears is the author of the best selling book, *The Zone.*

Too Much Carbohydrate

Over-carbing leads to excess insulin which leads to excess cortisol. And it all starts with too much of a good thing. Do you get sleepy after meals? Are you hungry within an hour or two after eating? Are you carrying any excess body fat? Then your body, which doesn't lie, is telling you that you're over-carbing. White carbs are the worst—white sugar, white flour, white bread. Try 40% protein, 40% good fat, and 20% good carbs.

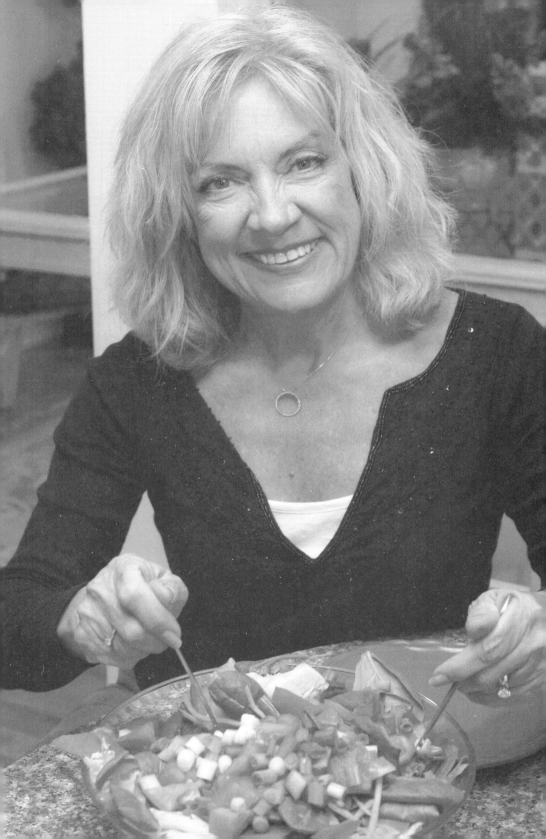

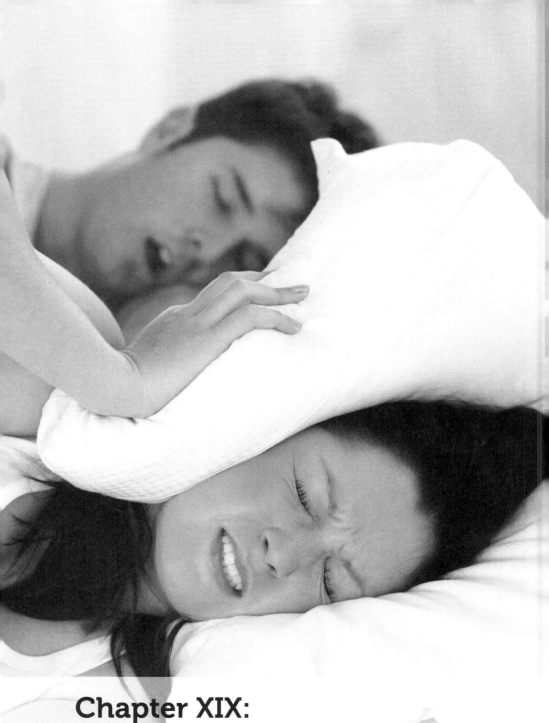

Chapter XIX:
Dental Sleep Medicine and
Sleep Disordered Breathing

Sleep Disordered Breathing ("SDB")

Obstructive Sleep Apnea ("OSA") and Dental Sleep Therapy

What are Sleep Disordered Breathing ("SDB") and Obstructive Sleep Apnea ("OSA")?

Many breathing changes can occur during sleep such as changes in frequency, depth, effectiveness, and sound; any such change which makes breathing more difficult or less effective is called Sleep Disordered Breathing or SDB.

Apnea ("without breath") is defined as lack of breathing. During sleep, this condition can take the form of either Obstructive Sleep Apnea ("OSA") caused by obstruction or blockage of the airway or Central Sleep Apnea ("CSA") caused by a decrease in the body's drive to breathe as regulated by the brain. Obstructive Sleep Apnea, characterized by muscle contractions in the attempt to breathe, can often be treated by the dentist, but Central Sleep Apnea, characterized by lack of attempt to breathe, and most other sleep disturbances, are treated by the physician and are outside the scope of our dental discussion.

What happens with Obstructive Sleep Apnea

Obstructive Sleep Apnea (OSA) occurs during sleep when the tongue and soft palate collapse onto the back of the throat, and the airway muscles relax so that they collapse inward and block the airway as the body attempts to breathe in.

Body trying to breathe in + airway collapse blocking airflow = OSA

Said differently, as we drop off to sleep, the muscles of the tongue and throat relax. When we attempt to breathe in, the tongue falls back and the airway walls get sucked in, together closing off the airway, and we

Snoring Can Kill You

Restoring sleep can save your alertness and your life!
The most important dental article you may ever read.

Sleep problems, as evidenced by snoring, interrupted breathing (apnea), and day time sleepiness can increase or cause:

- Snoring, gasping for breath, and restlessness during sleep
- Daytime sleepiness, fatigue, lack of energy, irritability
- Lack of focus, lack of concentration, inability to study
- Obesity, weight gain, eating for energy to stay awake
- Acting up, hyperactivity, "ADHD" (falsely diagnosed in kids)
- Increased blood pressure, heart problems, arteriosclerosis, kidney problems
- Disturbance of sleeping partner, marital problems
- Increased medical and pharmacy costs, "psychiatric" problems
- Auto accidents and work accidents

These problems are increased in women, especially with menopause, even more especially without hormone replacement therapy. In men, they are increased with age and weight.

Disturbed sleep breathing (obstructive sleep apnea) can act in the body like an injury, with tissue- de-oxygenation, releasing free radicals with damage to blood vessels. Adhesion factors are activated, causing build-up of arteriosclerotic plaques and narrowing of the arteries.

cannot then move air into the lungs. When the body's oxygen level drops low enough (oxygen deprivation), the drive to breathe increases until we partially awaken (an arousal), the airway muscles re-activate to open, the flow of air starts again (usually with a loud gasp), we breathe, and then fall back asleep. We usually do not remember these arousals when we later awaken.

This cycle of sleep, apnea, oxygen deprivation, arousal, airway opening, breath, and falling back to sleep repeats so you are never able to enter the deeper levels of sleep and never get the rest you need. You are deprived of the amount and depth of sleep you need, as well as the needed oxygen, so you are never truly rested and refreshed.

Snoring indicates airway problems. Silence then gasping for air indicates an apneic (airway blockage) episode followed by arousal with airway opening and breath. The harsh, noisy, breathing pattern of OSA, with snoring, snorting, gasping, grunting, and groaning adds to sleep disturbance of the bed partner and marital disharmony.

What are the numbers for Obstructive Sleep Apnea (OSA)?

Eighty percent of OSA patients are unaware of their condition. Yearly, almost forty thousand patients die because of an OSA-aggravated circulatory problem leading to heart attack or stroke.

Untreated OSA doubles your chance of dying within twelve years, and long-term untreated OSA increases the chance of dying young from an OSA-related medical problem by five times.

The AHI, Apnea-Hypopnea Index, is the number of times you stop breathing each hour of sleep.

- An AHI of less than 5 is considered normal, though zero (0) is ideal.

- An AHI of 5-15 is considered mild sleep apnea

- An AHI of 15-30 is considered moderate sleep apnea.

- An AHI greater than 30 is considered severe sleep apnea.

RDI, the Respiratory Disturbance Index, is the AHI (number of times you stop breathing per hour) plus the number of arousals per hour in an attempt to breathe, without full airway blockage and cessation of breathing. Your RDI will usually be higher than your AHI.

What are the signs and symptoms of OSA?

The combination of fragmented sleep and repeated episodes of oxygen deprivation (low oxygen levels) are the major contributors to the ill effects of Obstructive Sleep Apnea.

Lack of sleep results in EDS (Excessive Daytime Sleepiness), fatigue, lack of concentration, work-related accidents, driving-related accidents, lack of motivation, misdiagnosed "ADHD", Chronic Fatigue Syndrome, behavioral problems, psychiatric problems, and depression.

The periods of oxygen-deprivation contribute to heart attack, congestive heart failure, atherosclerosis, and other cardio-vascular problems. The repetitive hypoxias (oxygen deprivations) cause sympathetic (adrenalin-type) stimulation of the carotid bodies in the neck, resulting in hypertension (high blood pressure), kidney disease, stroke, and cardiac arrhythmias.

Newly-developed atrial fibrillation is often a function of Obstructive Sleep Apnea. OSA also contributes to GERD (gastro-esophageal reflux disease), ED (erectile dysfunction), TMJ, bruxism (tooth grinding), facial pain, headache, CFS (Chronic Fatigue Syndrome), over-eating, obesity, diabetes, and dementia.

Obstructive Sleep Apnea also appears to be highly related to Metabolic Syndrome, a combination of diabetes, insulin dysfunction, elevated cholesterol, elevated bad lipids, and high blood pressure. OSA and Sleep Disordered Breathing are causative factors in gestational (pregnancy) diabetes, gestational (pregnancy) hypertension, and fetal agitation. Pregnancy with snoring is often predictive of gestational hypertension. OSA is associated with increased rates of many types of cancer, including prostate cancer.

What are other medical problems related to OSA?

In the elderly, the effects of obstructive sleep apnea (attention deficit, delayed response time, memory loss, and decreased mental acuity) are often misinterpreted as dementia or Alzheimer's Disease. Use of nicotine, alcohol, caffeine, and many seemingly-innocuous medications can worsen OSA and worsen these effects.

Anti-depressants cause sedation in one-third of patients, and many of these are also OSA patients. These patients, even when successfully treated with CPAP (Continuous Positive Airway Pressure) or Oral Sleep Appliances for their OSA, may still be sleepy as a result of taking their anti-depressant. These medications may worsen the OSA and then mask the benefits of treatment.

Disruption of our normal circadian (24.2-hour night/day) pattern of sleep can also lessen the production of leptin, our satiety (eating-satisfaction) hormone, and increase production of ghrelin, our hunger-inducing hormone. OSA affects production of and sensitivity to insulin so the overall effect is increased eating and obesity which, in turn, worsens the sleep apnea. The increased body mass of obesity makes it more difficult to breathe in and thickens the fat pads in the neck and tongue, further closing down the airway and increasing the apnea. The cycle of increasing weight and worsening apnea continues. Our bodies operate in a circadian (actually 24.2 hour) cycle of night and day in which all body tissues follow the cycle which becomes compressed to match the 24 hour day. Hunger, alertness, body temperature, blood pressure, mood, and sleep-drive follow this cycle and become stressed and confused when disrupted by apnea and lack of sleep.

Human Growth Hormone is produced nightly during the deeper levels of sleep. Lack of these deep sleep levels disrupts HGH production and results in growth deficiency. Similarly, in males, testosterone production requires deep, regular, sleep. Sleep disruption can result in lack of testosterone during the critical growth years and as we age.

What are the risk factors for (causes of) SDB (Sleep Disordered Breathing) and OSA?

Increased age, weight, obesity, sleeping on the back, male gender, snoring, and thick neck increase the risk for SDB and OSA. In Obesity-Hypoventilation Syndrome, the mass of the body tissues and thickness of the neck decrease the ability of the patient to fully draw breath. Similarly, alcohol prior to sleep, Viagra-type medications, narcotic pain medications, and sedatives increase the OSA risk.

What about age?

SDB and OSA are most commonly problems of increasing age, and worsen as we get older, but are also found in young children (as early as infancy and adolescence) and may be experienced at any age. SDB and OSA in young children, are often indicators of current airway problems and predictors of future sleep apnea and developmental problems.

Deep regular sleep helps insure proper production of Human Growth Hormone, and, in males, of testosterone. Future "TMJ" or "TMD" problems are often caused by airway obstruction during facial development. Airway problems in kids should be corrected to aid in proper sleep, normal growth, and avoidance of future "TMJ" problems.

What about snoring?

Snoring is indicative of airway problems and is the result of vibration of the soft tissues of the throat (usually the soft palate and uvula). It is caused by uneven or obstructed air flow during sleep, and it may be soft and pleasant or loud and annoying. Snoring with silence and then gasping is indicative of sleep apnea (obstructed airflow) and then restart of breathing. Snoring (even "benign" snoring) creates vibrations in the upper airway which damage the upper airway neurons (nerves) and muscles, causing decreased airway neuro-muscular reflex, decreased airway dilator muscle function (not totally reversible, even with treatment), impaired dilator reflex, and upper airway collapse during sleep.

- Snoring vibration
  - ⟹ Demyelination (damage) of airway muscle nerves
    - ⟹ Decreased function of airway dilator muscles
      - ⟹ Obstructive Sleep Apnea

Snoring can cause progressive OSA with the damage irreversible, even with treatment. Early treatment for snoring and apnea can lessen future apnea and sleep-disordered breathing problems. Pediatric tonsil/adenoid problems and snoring are diagnostic of SDB and predictive of future OSA. Treatment of pediatric airway problems, including removal of tonsils and adenoids and treatment of nasal congestion, should not wait until "they grow out of it," as delayed treatment can result in continued airway problems, changes in the growth of the jaws and face, and physiologic problems which prevent proper body growth and intellectual development.

Again, proper production of Human Growth Hormone and testosterone require deep, regular sleep during these critical formative years. So correction of adolescent airway problems aids normal physical and intellectual development. Normal airway and sleep also promote proper facial growth and avoidance of future "TMJ" and facial pain problems.

Should I treat my snoring?

Snoring should never be treated without the same medical sleep work-up indicated for OSA; evaluation by a qualified sleep physician and polysomnography ("PSG", a full sleep study to evaluate the body's physical state as it relates to sleep). Prior to treatment for snoring, the physician should rule out the presence of Obstructive Sleep Apnea because it is possible for an apneic and snoring patient to mistakenly assume that only snoring is present and to only desire treatment for the snoring. In such a case, the noisy (snoring) apnic, treated only for the snoring, becomes a silent apnic with no recognized symptoms of the apnea. A noisy (snoring) apnic is recognizable and treatable; a silent apnic may go undiagnosed, and this can be deadly. Only if no OSA is present should snoring alone be the focus of oral sleep appliance therapy.

Similarly, in oral sleep appliance therapy, snoring is often eliminated prior to the apnea. Elimination of the snoring, though a nice bonus, is never an indicator of successful treatment for sleep apnea.

What about OSA and insomnia?

Sleep apnea and insomnia are often similar and associated but not identical. Obstructive sleep apnea is the unsuccessful attempt to breathe in, despite airway blockage. Insomnia is the inability to fall asleep or stay asleep, independent of the above-noted physical causes. If both OSA and insomnia are present, the sleep deprivation is made worse, and both are under-estimated when the other is present. The OSA patient cannot breathe in and is helped by CPAP therapy and/or oral appliance therapy; the insomniac can often not tolerate either of the therapies. If the patient has both OSA and insomnia, he or she often cannot tolerate the best available therapies. Facial surgery to move the jaws forward and open the airway may be the only answer.

What is the relation between leg edema, neck edema, and SDB/OSA?

Those with leg edema (fluid accumulation and swelling) are much more likely to suffer from nighttime breathing problems. Patients with leg edema accumulate fluid in the legs daily as the result of sitting for long periods (muscle function not being active to help "pump" fluids back up to the heart), obesity, congestive heart failure, and salt intake. Upon lying down, this excess fluid is redistributed throughout the body, especially into the neck, causing upper airway edema (swelling), compression of the airway, and aggravation of airway problems (OSA). Preventing this daily leg edema and the resultant nightly airway problems involves daily exercise, not sitting for long periods, use of compression stockings, decreased salt intake, diuretics, and treatment of the underlying heart failure. CPAP or Oral Appliance therapies can then be more effective.

What about Gastro-Esophageal Reflux (GER) or Gastro-Esophageal Reflux Disease (GERD)?

GERD can cause rapid destruction of the teeth as well as severe medical problems and is intimately related to OSA. GERD is the result of relaxation of the sphincter (valve) between the esophagus and the stomach, allowing escape of stomach acid into the esophagus, throat, mouth, and possibly the lungs (Pulmonary Aspiration). Possible results are esophagitis, laryngitis, pharyngitis, acid erosion of the teeth, and asthma.

At night, with the body sleeping and horizontal, the sphincter relaxes and allows increased volume of stomach acid into the esophagus. With little saliva produced and less swallowing during sleep, there is slow clearing of the acid and heightened potential for acid damage.

During the apneic periods of OSA, the muscles of the chest and abdomen strain to breathe, and this helps to expel more stomach acid. In the horizontal position of sleep, more acid reaches the upper esophagus and airway.

GERD occurs in 70% of OSA patients; the exact cause and effect relationship is unclear, but the association is proven. If the GERD is treated, then the OSA may improve; if the OSA is treated, then the GERD may improve. The individual results are highly variable, but both conditions must be treated for maximum patient benefit.

How is Obstructive Sleep Apnea Diagnosed?

Since OSA is a serious medical condition, it must be diagnosed by a physician with full patient history and examination. Diagnosis is based on the results of an overnight sleep study, called a Polysomnogram (PSG), which records breathing, heart rate, blood oxygenation, muscle activity, EEG (brain activity), EKG (heart activity), position, and other physical parameters. This sleep study may be performed either in a sleep lab or at home. An in-lab PSG has the advantage of more channels of information for the physician to use in his or her diagnosis, more video and audio information recorded, and immediate correction of errors by the on-site sleep technician.

The disadvantage of the in-lab study is in the "first night effect" that often results in the patient not achieving a normal night's sleep due to lack of comfort in a different bed and unfamiliar surroundings.

An in-home study uses a simpler sleep monitoring system that supplies fewer channels of physiologic data with which the physician can diagnose your sleep issues, but often has the advantage of the patient's own bed, familiar surroundings, familiar bed partner, and a better night's sleep. This better night's sleep may then give more accurate sleep information, which is more indicative of the usual night's sleep pattern.

Are all sleep problems the result of airway problems?

There are many medical sleep disorders for which airway obstruction is not the cause.

There is a difference between Sleep-Disordered Breathing (SDB) and disordered sleep due to poor sleep habits and poor sleep preparation (sleep hygiene). Many sleep problems have no relationship to airway problems, and they require complex medical evaluation, diagnosis, and treatment. CPAP and oral sleep appliances will not correct problems with the central (brain) drive to breathe. In these cases of hypoventilation (decreased breathing) caused by Central Sleep Apnea (decreased drive to breathe) and in other medically-caused sleep breathing problems, CPAP and oral sleep appliances may play an adjunctive role after the underlying medical problems have been diagnosed and treated. Oral sleep appliances alone can not treat many of the breathing problems of age, obesity, smoking, COPD, heart failure, partial muscle paralysis, reduced lung capacity, cancer, and narcotic abuse because airway is not the problem.

Restless Leg Syndrome, Periodic Limb Movement Disorder, and Sleep-Onset (circadian rhythm) disorders are also medical disorders requiring physician diagnosis and treatment prior to any oral appliance therapy.

Once diagnosed, what are the treatment options for OSA (airway) problems?

Once diagnosed with OSA, patients may elect better sleep hygiene (habits), weight loss, exercise, and change in sleep position (not on the back). They may elect to avoid alcohol, narcotics, Viagra, and sedatives prior to sleep. Medical and dental treatments include Continuous Positive Airway Pressure (CPAP), Oral Sleep Appliances, and Nasal Air Valves (Provent). Nightly airway problems may be helped with medical treatment of leg edema, GERD, heart problems, diabetes, upper airway resistance (UAR), and nasal congestion.

In cases where CPAP and Oral Sleep Appliances are not effective or tolerated by the patient (due to limiting factors such as claustrophobia or insomnia), then surgery may be required to expand the airway by advancing (moving forward) the upper and lower jaws.

What is Continuous Positive Airway Pressure (CPAP) and how does it work for treating OSA?

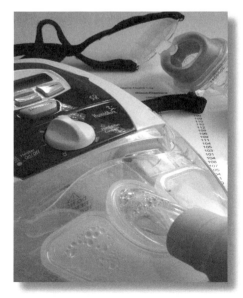

Continuous Positive Airway Pressure (CPAP) is pressurized air generated from a bedside machine. The air is delivered though a tube, connected to a mask which covers the nose and mouth, and the force of the pressurized air gently keeps the airway open. CPAP opens the airway just as air does when blown into a balloon; it opens and expands, and this is exactly how CPAP clears the airway. CPAP is the "gold standard" of OSA treatment and provides the best treatment results. However, many patients have problems with mask fit, mask leaks, facial irritation, and pump noise. They may also be disturbed by movement restriction, facial straps, drying of the airway, machine noise, or general discomfort. Though CPAP is more highly effective, dental sleep appliances have greater compliance (use) and are indicated in those OSA patients intolerant of CPAP.

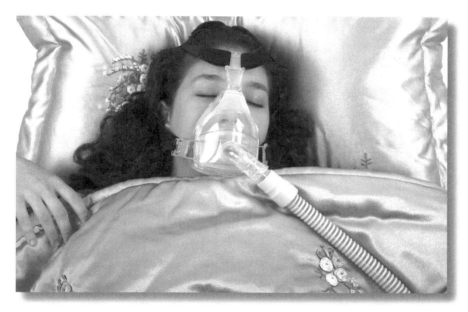

What About Oral Sleep Appliance Therapy?

Oral sleep appliances are worn in the mouth to treat snoring and OSA. These devices are similar to orthodontic retainers or sports mouth guards. Oral Sleep Appliance Therapy involves the selection, design, fitting, and use of a custom-designed oral appliance that is worn during sleep, and this appliance then attempts to maintain an opened, unobstructed airway in the throat. There are many different oral appliances available. Well over 100 appliances have been approved through the FDA for treatment of snoring and/or Sleep Apnea. Oral appliances may be used alone or in combination with other means of treating OSA, including improved sleep hygiene, weight management, surgery, and CPAP.

Oral Appliances work in several ways:

- Repositioning and holding the tongue forward to open the airway

- Repositioning the tongue, soft palate, and uvula to open the airway

- Repositioning the lower jaw forward to then hold the tongue forward to open the airway

- Stabilizing the lower jaw and tongue forward to open the airway

- Increasing the muscle tone of the tongue and throat muscles to dilate (open) the airway

Dentists with training in Oral Sleep Appliance Therapy are familiar with the various designs of appliances and can determine which one is best suited for your needs. We will work with your physician as part of the medical team in your diagnosis, treatment, and on-going care.

Can dentistry help you and your bed partner?

Snoring, groaning, gasping, and excessive moving during sleep can also disturb the sleep of your bed partner and those sleeping nearby. Loud snoring by one member has been known to keep awake entire families. Certainly, one partner or spouse kept awake by the other's snoring does not make for a rested partner, harmonious relationships, or a happy household.

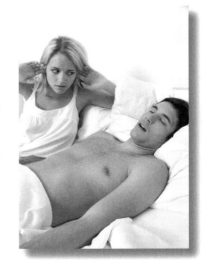

Oral Sleep Appliance Therapy can help you obtain the rest you need, your bed partner the quiet he or she desires, and your relationship the harmony it deserves.

I Have TMJ.
Can I still use an Oral Sleep Appliance?

These appliances can be used by patients with TMJ and muscle problems of the face. Care must be taken to titrate (adjust) the appliance slowly to the effective position, and the morning exercises must be performed conscientiously to reseat the TMJ's (jaw joints) and reprogram (relax) the jaw muscles. Any TMD/TMJ symptoms are usually transient (short-term) and improve with time, special exercises, hot soaks (e.g. hot towels) on the muscles with exercises, and possible anti-inflammatory medications such as ibuprofen. Occasionally, we may need to modify the appliance to decrease nightly muscle activity or change appliances, possibly using a tongue-retaining device instead of our standard mandibular-advancement device.

What are the steps involved in Oral Sleep Appliance Therapy?

1. Medical Consultation for your sleep problems

2. Sleep Study (Polysomnogram, PSG)

3. Final medical diagnosis leading to confirmation of obstructive sleep apnea

4. CPAP consideration, evaluation, and possible use

5. CPAP re-evaluation; if refused or not tolerated, then physician referral to qualified sleep dentist for oral sleep appliance

6. Dental evaluation of oral structures and oral health to insure suitability of Oral Sleep Appliance Therapy

7. Review of possible side effects and long-term changes in bite, muscles, tooth position, and jaw position due to Oral Sleep Appliance Therapy

8. Review of the need for exercises to reposition the jaw each morning after appliance wear to minimize the speed and extent of long-term bite and jaw changes. These exercises may involve biting into a morning jaw-repositioning appliance and/or gently pushing the jaw backward into its correct position with your hand and arm for some minutes each morning.

9. Full review of informed consent for Oral Sleep Appliance Therapy

10. Determination of the proper oral appliance for you

11. Impressions of the upper and lower teeth for appliance fabrication

12. Determination of the proper jaw and tongue position to open the airway at the initial treatment position

13. Special bite registration of the jaws in the initial treatment position

14. Fabrication and delivery of the sleep appliance (usually two-four weeks later)

15. Review of instructions for appliance use and titration (adjustment) by the patient

16. Review of instructions for sleep-monitoring device, if used

17. Titration (adjustment) of appliance by patient to effective sleep position determined by:

    a. Relief of sleep-deprivation symptoms

    b. Decrease in daily sleepiness

    c. Reports from bed partner

    d. Results from sleep monitor, if used

18. Handling of any side-effects or problems

19. Continued morning exercises to reposition the jaw and minimize tooth, joint, and muscle changes

20. Determination/adjustment of appliance position for most effective sleep jaw position

21. Finalization of appliance and jaw position with home sleep monitor

22. Follow-up sleep study (PSG) with the sleep physician and confirmation of appliance effectiveness at current position

23. Stabilization of oral sleep appliance, as necessary, at the final position

24. Scheduling of regular follow-up visits with the sleep dentist to handle appliance therapy side effects, complications, or other long-term considerations

Some considerations For Oral Sleep Appliance Therapy

Custom (dentist-made) oral appliances are much safer and more effective than over-the-counter "boil-and-bite" sleep appliances, which are much less effective initially and much, much, less effective over time. These store-bought sleep appliances can not be used to determine if oral sleep appliance therapy will work for you, as they can over-open the jaw, decrease the airway opening, and give inconsistent results.

Custom-made, adjustable appliances work best. There are sometimes trade-offs between effectiveness and (initial) comfort; the patient may need to weigh adaptability to the appliance vs. maximum effectiveness.

Long-term results are not based on the results of a single night's use because of the variables of sleep hygiene, nasal congestion, leg edema, exercise, and one night's possible disturbances. Appliance therapy is based on long-term treatment effectiveness, long-term comfort, and long-term minimal side-effects. If one expects improved health, feeling better, less fatigue, and less snoring, then oral sleep appliance therapy is a good choice. If one expects absolute elimination of OSA episodes, then CPAP is the best choice. There is no "correct" choice between CPAP and Oral Sleep Appliance Therapy; each has its own set of considerations; and the therapy must be matched to patient preference.

If one chooses Oral Sleep Appliance Therapy, then the best choice is a custom-made, titrateable (adjustable), movable (not fixed) appliance that minimally opens the bite. Many such appliances are available, and the choice of which one to use is based on patient preference, comfort, long-term effectiveness, and long-term minimal side-effects.

Our goal for you in dental sleep medicine is good sleep, good days, good health, and long life.

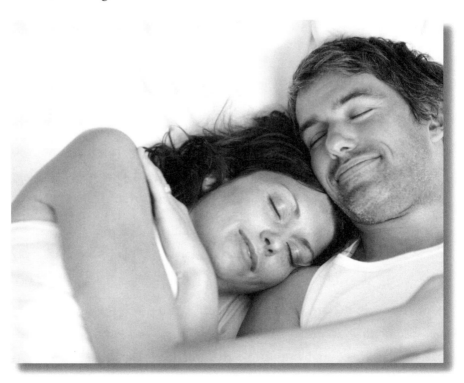

Silent Night for Snorers

"Laugh and the whole world laughs with you; snore and you sleep alone."

Anti-snoring devices may restore domestic tranquility and ensure a good night's sleep to the families and friends of people who snore. Snoring can be defined as rough, noisy breathing caused by vibration of the uvula, which looks like a bell clapper at the back of the throat, and the soft palate, which is the soft tissue just beyond the roof of your mouth This noisy nighttime habit affects an estimated 20 million to 60 million Americans.

One simple remedy is to sew a marble into a pocket on the back of the pajama tops to discourage sleeping on the back. But for many snorers, the answer is not that simple.

Attempts to solve a snoring problem include surgical removal of some of the soft palate, a tongue- retaining device and a sound-activated awakening device. There are more than 300 anti-snoring devices registered in the United States patent office. Dentists sometimes prescribe such a device for a patient, usually in consultation with a sleep clinic. Treatment for snoring first requires a sleep study to rule out sleep apnea, a much more deadly affliction.

Obesity contributes to the problem by increasing the width and build of the oral tissues. High stress levels, consuming large quantities of alcohol, and sleeping on the back might also induce snoring.

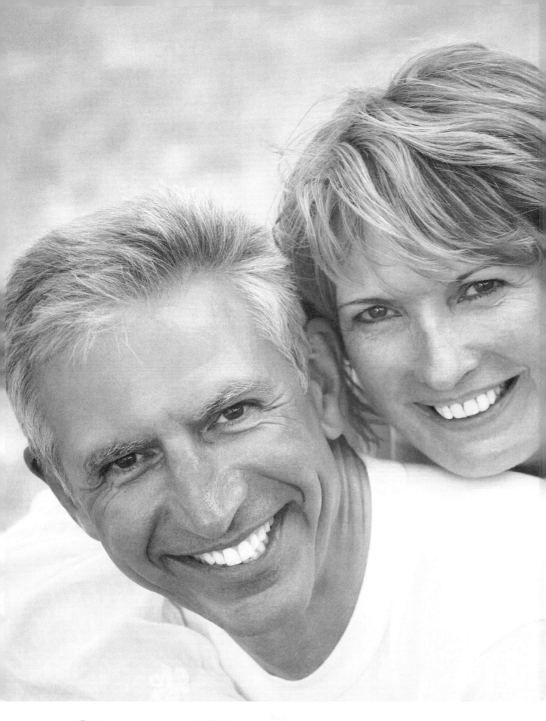

Chapter XX:
Relax!

Relaxing in Dentistry and in Life

If you are scared of being in the dental chair and get upset at the mere thought of your dental visit, we can help you relax. We always recommend that relationship, communication, and trust be the foundation for a comfortable dental visit. Knowing that we can be trusted to care for you like family and to always put your comfort and care first are the beginning of relaxing comfort dentistry.

However, the dental chair is not the only place where relaxation is a good thing. There are many things you can do to help you relax and reduce stress in other areas of life.

52 Proven Stress Reducers from the National Headache Foundation
To protect your cardiac and mental health

1. Get up fifteen minutes earlier in the morning. The inevitable morning mishaps will be less stressful.

2. Prepare for the morning the evening before. Set the breakfast table, make lunches, put out the clothes to plan to wear, etc.

3. Don't rely on your memory. Write down appointment times, when to pick up the laundry, when library books are due, etc. ("The palest ink is better than the most retentive memory"- Old Chinese Proverb)

4. Do nothing which, after being done, leads you to tell a lie.

5. Make duplicates of all keys. Bury a house key in a secret spot in the garden and carry a duplicate car key in your wallet, apart from your key ring.

6. Practice preventative maintenance. Your car, appliances, home, and relationships will be less likely to break down/ fall apart "at the worst possible moment."

7. Be prepared to wait. A paperback can make a wait in a post office line almost pleasant.

8. Procrastination is stressful. Whatever you want to do tomorrow, do today; whatever you want to do today, do it now.

9. Plan ahead. Don't let the gas tank fall below one-quarter full; keep a well-stocked "emergency shelf" of home staples; don't wait until you're down to your last bus token or postage stamp to buy more.

10. Don't put up with something that doesn't work right. If your alarm clock, wallet, shoe laces, windshield wipers—whatever—are a constant aggravation, get them fixed or get new ones.

11. Allow 15 minutes extra time to get to appointments. Plan to arrive at an airport one hour before domestic departures.

12. Eliminate (or restrict) the amount of caffeine in your diet.

13. Always set up contingency plans, "just in case." ("If for some reason either of us is delayed, here's what we'll do..." kind of thing. Or, "If we get split up in the shopping center, here's where we'll meet.")

14. Relax your standards. The world will not end if the grass doesn't get mowed this weekend.

15. Pollyanna-Power! For every one thing that goes wrong, there are probably 10 or 50 or 100 blessings; count 'em!

16. Ask questions. Taking a few moments to repeat back directions, what someone expects of you, etc., can save hours. (The old "the hurrieder I go, the behinder I get" idea).

17. Say "No!" Say "no" to extra projects, social activities, and invitations you know you don't have the time or energy for. This takes self-respect and a belief that everyone, everyday, needs quiet time to relax and be alone.

18. Unplug your phone. Want to take a long bath, meditate, sleep, or read without interruption? Drum up the courage to temporarily

disconnect. (The possibility of there being a terrible emergency in the next hour or so is almost nil.)

19. Turn "needs" into preferences. Our basic physical needs translate into food, water, and keeping warm. Everything else is a preference. Don't get attached to preferences.

20. Simplify, simplify, simplify...

21. Make friends with non-worriers. Nothing can get you into the habit of worrying faster than associating with chronic worrywarts.

22. Get up and stretch periodically if your job requires you sit for extended periods of time.

23. Wear earplugs. If you need to find quiet at home, pop in some earplugs.

24. Get enough sleep. If necessary, use an alarm clock to remind you to go to bed.

25. Create order out of chaos. Organize your home and workspace so that you can always know exactly where things are. Put things away where they belong, and you won't have to go through the stress of losing things.

26. When feeling stressed, most people tend to breathe in short, shallow breaths. When you breathe like this, stale air is not expelled, oxidation of the tissues is incomplete, and muscle tension frequently results. Check your breathing throughout the day and before, during, and after high pressure situations. If you find your stomach muscles are knotted and your breathing is shallow, relax all your muscles and take several deep, slow breaths. Note how, when you're relaxed, both your abdomen and chest expand when you breathe.

27. Writing your thoughts and feelings down (in a journal or on paper to be thrown away) can help clarify things and can give you a renewed perspective.

28. Try the following yoga technique whenever you feel the need to relax. Inhale deeply through your nose to the count of eight. Then, with lips puckered, exhale very slowly through your mouth to the count of 16, or for as long as you can. Concentrate on the long sighing sound and feel the tension dissolve. Repeat 10 times.

29. Inoculate yourself against a feared event. Example: Before speaking in public, take time to go over every part of the experience in your mind. Imagine what you'll wear, what the audience will look like, how you will present your talk, what the questions will be, how you will answer them, etc. Visualize the experience the way you would have it be. You will likely find that when the time comes to make the actual presentation, it will be "old hat" and much of your anxiety will have fled.

30. When the stress of having to get a job done gets in the way of getting the job done, diversion- a voluntary change in activity and/ or environment—may be just what you need. Then reward yourself with a short, timed reward for each hour of work on your project.

31. Talk it out. Discussing your problems with a trusted friend can help clear your mind of confusion so you can concentrate on problem solving.

32. One of the most obvious ways to avoid unnecessary stress is to select an environment (work, home, leisure) which is in line with your personal needs and desires. If you hate desk jobs, don't accept a job which requires that you sit at a desk all day. If you hate to talk politics, don't associate with people who love to talk politics, etc.

33. Learn to live one day at a time.

34. Every day, do something you really enjoy.

35. Add an ounce of love to everything you do.

36. Take a hot bath or shower (or cool one in summertime) to relieve tension.

37. Do something for somebody else.

    "If you want others to be happy, practice compassion. If you want to be happy, practice compassion." - *The Dalai Lama*

38. Focus on understanding rather than on being understood; on loving rather than being loved. ("Be interested, not interesting.")

39. Do something that will improve your appearance. Looking better can help you feel better.

40. Schedule a realistic day. Avoid the tendency to schedule back-to-back appointments; allow time between appointments for a breathing spell.

41. Become more flexible. Some things are worth not doing perfectly and some issues are well to compromise on.

42. Eliminate destructive self-talk: "I'm too old to...," "I'm too fat to....," etc.

43. Use your weekend time for change of pace. If your work week is slow and patterned, make sure there is action and time for spontaneity built into your weekends. If your work week is fast-paced and full of people and deadlines, seek peace and solitude during your days off. Feel as if you aren't accomplishing anything at work? Tackle a job on the weekend which you can finish to your satisfaction.

44. "Worry about the pennies and the dollars will take care of themselves." That's another way of saying: take care of todays as best you can and the yesterdays and the tomorrows will take care of themselves.

45. Do one thing at a time. When you are with someone, be with that person and with no one and nothing else. When you are busy with a project, concentrate on doing that project and forget about everything else you have to do.

46. Allow yourself time-everyday- for privacy, quiet, and introspection.

47. If you face an especially unpleasant task, do it early in the day and get it over with; then the rest of the day will be free of anxiety.

48. Learn to delegate responsibilities to capable others.

49. Don't forget to take a lunch break. Try to get away from your desk or work area in body and mind, even if it's just for 15 or 20 minutes.

50. Forget about counting to 10. Count to 1000 before doing something or saying anything that could make matters worse. You cannot unring a bell or take back those words once spoken.

51. Have a forgiving view of events and people. Accept the fact that we live in an imperfect world.

52. Have an optimistic view of the world. Believe that most people are doing the best they can with who they are and what they know.

Travel Tips:
Handling out-of-town Dental Emergencies

Pack a dental emergency kit next to your cruisewear and sunscreen before heading our for vacation this year.

A toothache, lost filling, or broken retainer needn't spoil your fun away from home as long as you've got the basics of dental first-aid in your suitcase: oil of cloves, aspirin or aspirin substitutes, bicarbonate of soda, gauze pads, cotton swabs, floss, and paraffin (wax).

Remember, your dental first-aid kit is intended for temporary emergency care before you can find your way to a dentist or hospital emergency room. If you're in the US, and you need a dentist, contact the local dental society. If you're out of the country, contact the US embassy or ask the hotel personnel to refer you. If you're out in the wilderness and the nearest town is 100 miles away—all the more reason to have a dental first aid kit in your gear!

Follow these instructions:

- **Toothache or sore and injured area:** Rinse your mouth vigorously with warm water to clean out debris. You might also try rinsing with a mild solution of salt and warm water. Use floss to remove any food that might be trapped between teeth.

If swelling is present, place cold compresses on the outside of the cheek. Do not use heat and do not place aspirin on the gum tissue or aching tooth.

- **Knocked-out tooth:** Place the tooth in cold milk (best), contact lens saline, or cold water. Do not scrub the tooth. Or, you can reposition the tooth, handling it as little as possible. Rinse your mouth first with a solution of water and bicarbonate of soda. See a dentist immediately; lost teeth can sometimes be re-implanted.

- **Lost filling:** Apply oil of cloves to cotton. Squeeze out the excess and place a small piece of cotton in the cavity with paraffin (wax). Take aspirin as needed.

- **Bitten tongue or lip:** Apply direct pressure with a clean cloth. Apply cold compresses. If bleeding doesn't stop, or if the bite is severe, head to a dentist or hospital emergency room.

- **Objects wedged between teeth:** Remove the object with floss. Don't use sharp or pointed instruments.

- **Orthodontic problems:** If a wire is causing irritation, cover the end with a small cotton ball, a piece of gauze, or wax. If the wire is embedded in the cheek, tongue, or gum; do not try to take it out. Save any loose or broken pieces of wire and take them with you to the dentist or orthodontist.

- **Possible jaw fracture:** Immobilize the jaw by any means (e.g., with a handkerchief, tie, towel) and go to a hospital emergency room.

- **Cold sore (Herpes Labialis):** Apply ice for 30 minutes, take Lysine 1000 mg three to four times daily, avoid Arginine (in chocolate and nuts), and apply Abreva (over-the-counter).

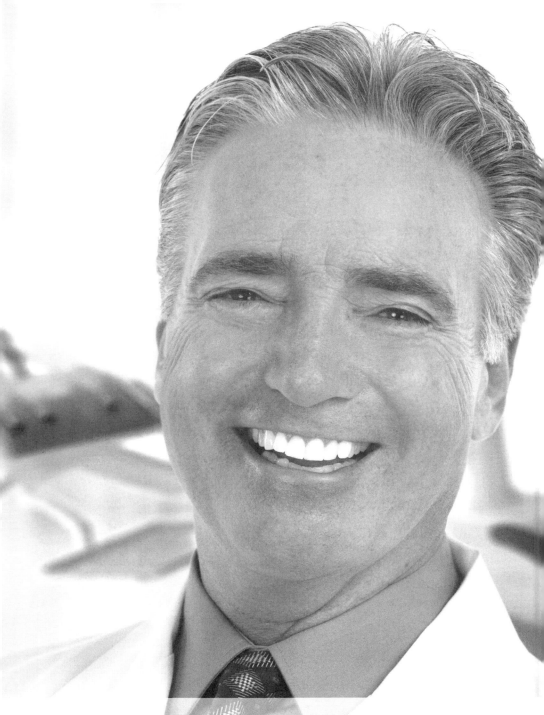

Chapter XXII:
The Oral-Systemic Connection

The Oral-Systemic Connection

How Oral (Dental) Health Affects Systemic (Medical) Health

A White Paper for Physicians, Dentists, and Patients
By
Robert A. Finkel, DDS, MAGD, FICCMO, FACMS

Restorative and Cosmetic Dentistry
for a Healthy Natural Smile
Temporomandibular Disorders and Dental Sleep Medicine

Suggested Additional Readings following

Table of Contents:

A. Introduction

Only recently have the medical and dental professions realized the intimate connection between oral (dental) health and systemic (medical) health. Miller's "Focal Theory of Infection" (pub. 1891), popular in the early 1900's, held that cavities, periodontal (gum) disease, and dental infections could have long-ranging effects and could cause systemic disease in other organ systems of the body. This concept lost credence and was thoroughly denounced even into the 1980's.

Since the 1990's, evidence has been heavily mounting that there is, indeed, an oral-systemic connection, and that compromised oral health is associated with compromised systemic health. The mature biofilm of periodontal infection stimulates a strong local inflammatory response and allows bacteria and bacterial by-products to enter the bloodstream. It turns out that Miller's 1891 Focal Theory of Infection may be real, causing foci of inflammation and/or infection in distant body systems.

Oral disease has been associated with cardio-vascular disease, heart attack, stroke, Metabolic Disorder, diabetes, complications of pregnancy, kidney disease, cancer, and respiratory illness. Conversely, oral health has been associated with lessened risk of these conditions. Following is more detailed information about these associations, and how treatment of oral disease improves systemic health outcomes; how working in partnership with the physician, dentists can contribute to the health, longevity, and well-being of our patients.

B. Connection Between Periodontal Disease and C-Reactive Protein (CRP)

Medical evidence has now established connections between oral infection, the resultant inflammation, and distant inflammatory disease. Death and phagocytosis of oral bacteria (especially gram-negative bacteria) cause formation and release of endotoxins, cytokines, and various groups of immune and inflammatory up-regulators. The various cytokines involved in feedback loops, the coagulation pathway, and the compliment pathway contribute to acute and chronic inflammation, and cause the liver to produce C-Reactive Protein (CRP). hs-CRP levels are a strong indicator of a future cardiovascular event, and current evidence indicates that CRP levels are an indicator of ongoing inflammation, a predictor of future inflammatory disease occurance, and likely a contributing factor to those ongoing disease processes. Periodontal therapy can decrease CRP levels. Pre-treatment and post-treatment CRP levels should be measured and the level is often seen to drop after our periodontal therapy.

C. Periodontitis and Cardiac Disease

Inflammation, up-regulated by periodontal disease, is the major oral-systemic connection, and systemic inflammation is the silent killer. Periodontal disease is a medical problem with a dental solution.

The "old" view of cardiovascular disease is that of athero-sclerotic plaques "clogging the pipes" of the arteries; narrowing the arteries and obstructing arterial blood flow. Inflammation is now seen as a major factor in atherosclerosis. Inflammation increases oxidation of LDL, increasing fatty plaque in the vessel wall, and thinning of the epithelial lining. These fatty plaques can calcify and further narrow the arterial lumen, or they can rupture and initiate a blood clot, occluding the lumen, and initiating an infarct of the downstream tissues. Dental disease increases the circulating levels of fibrinogen and white blood cells. Oral bacteria are also found in the atherosclerotic lesions and thrombi, indicating that infection in these arteries is a component of the disease, either directly or as a result, again, of the inflammatory process.

Studies show a strong statistical link between poor oral hygiene, poor dental (periodontal) health, and cardiovascular disease. Patients with heart attack, stroke, and EKG changes have, by study and statistics, higher levels of periodontal disease and the resultant inflammatory burden.

D. Periodontitis and Stroke

As noted above, studies indicate a strong correlation between the infection and inflammation of periodontal disease. Poor oral hygiene and periodontal disease are risk factors for a CVA stroke involving ischemia or blockage of cerebral blood vessels.

The infectious/inflammatory process outlined above involving the cytokine pathways, coagulation pathways, and compliment pathways can cause equivalent damage in both the cardiac and cranial vessels. Treatment of periodontal disease and improved periodontal health are correlated with lessened risk of ischemic stroke.

E. Periodontitis and Pregnancy

Periodontitis and its related inflammation have been shown to be associated with pre-term delivery and low birth-weight infants. Studies indicate that periodontal infection can lead to placental-fetal inflammatory exposure and fetal inflammation, resulting in pre-term delivery. Pre-term infants face a higher risk of neurological, respiratory, and behavioral problems, learning disabilities, and metabolic abnormalities. Studies also indicate that periodontal infection may have deleterious effects on the growth and development of the fetus and infant, in addition to those caused by pre-term delivery.

Pregnancy complications are associated with the inflammatory factors of systemic, urinary tract, and periodontal infections. Pregnancy complications are shown to be highly associated with higher CRP and cytokine levels associated with periodontal pathogens. The inflammatory mediators may cross the placental barrier, causing fetal development deformities and loss of viability.

While we do not know if treating periodontal disease in pregnant women will improve pregnancy outcomes, we do know that periodontal health is associated with improved pregnancy outcomes and improved fetal health.

F. Obesity and Diabetes

Studies have shown a strong correlation between periodontal disease and obesity, and that the incidence of periodontitis is 76% higher in obese young adults. Excess adipose tissue actually secrets a variety of cytokines and hormones involved in the inflammatory process, and periodontal disease shares many of the same inflammatory pathways. The adipokines (leptin, resistin, and adiponectin) are active players in the body's inflammatory response and may aggravate the immunological side-effects of periodontal disease. Similarly, the inflammatory mediators of periodontal disease may aggravate the factors leading to obesity.

Periodontal disease is also highly associated with Diabetes and Metabolic Disorder, and studies indicate that patients with periodontal disease have greater difficulty in controlling their blood sugar levels.

The inflammation of periodontal disease appears to be a major contributor to the pathogenesis, complications, and poor metabolic control of diabetes. The metabolic and inflammatory pathways initiated by the periodontal infection appear to adversely affect pancreatic beta-cell health, insulin-resistance, blood-sugar control, and HgA1c levels. Periodontal infection also increases the incidence and severity of Metabolic Syndrome (obesity, lipid abnormalities, hypertension, hyperglycemia, diabetes/insulin disorder). Metabolic Syndrome appears to be worsened by the inflammation of periodontal disease and the formation of Advanced Glycation End-products (AGEs) during periods of hyperglycemia and oxidative stress. These and other inflammatory mediators are shown to cause tissue destruction associated with Diabetes and Metabolic Syndrome. Treatment of periodontal disease is improved with proper treatment of diabetes, and diabetes treatment improves periodontal outcomes.

G. Kidney Disease

Chronic Kidney Disease (CKD) is more common in adults who are partially or fully edentulous. Research suggests that the same inflammatory response which causes the bone loss and tooth loss of periodontal disease also causes the damage of CKD.

Adults with tooth loss and periodontal disease have twice the incidence of kidney disease; overlapping inflammatory pathways are the common factor.

H. Respiratory Problems and Lung Disease

Recent research implicates the mouth and throat as sources of respiratory infections. Normal oral bacteria can be aspirated and cause lung infections; this appears to be increased in the presence of periodontal infection and resultant increase in the number and types of pathogenic bacteria present. Chronic Obstructive Pulmonary Disease (COPD) also decreases the clearance of bacteria from the lungs and increases the severity of the problem. Lung disease is correlated with the clinical, bacterial, and inflammatory markers of periodontal disease. Periodontal disease inflammatory pathways, outlined previously, may also initiate and aggravate inflammation and swelling of the lung tissues.

I. Cancer

Statistically, patients with periodontal disease have a 63% increase in pancreatic cancer, 33-36% increase in lung cancer, 50% increase in kidney cancer, and a 30+% increase in blood cell cancers. Head and neck cancers are much more common in patients with periodontal disease, and men with periodontal disease showed a 14% overall increase in cancer rates. University studies also show a correlation between H. pylori (possibly of oral origin) and stomach cancer. Incidentally, Human Papilloma Virus (HPV), when found orally and genitally is a strong predictor/cause of oral and cervical cancers.

J. Osteoporosis

University studies show a link between periodontal disease and osteoporosis. The low bone density of osteoporosis is definitely associated with periodontal bone loss and tooth loss; all increase with advancing age, though the correlation is independent of age. Tooth loss from periodontal disease correlates with menopause in women, osteopenia (decreased bone density and possible precursor to osteoporosis), use of oral contraceptives, and increased periodontal infection.

Treatments for osteoporosis include decreased use of birth control pills, post-menopausal hormone replacement therapy, calcium/vitamin D therapy, and dental periodontal therapy. Oral therapy includes dental scaling to remove bacterial deposits, hygiene-access surgery, localized antibiotic therapy, and systemic drug therapy. Research is ongoing to determine the cause and effect relationship between osteoporosis and periodontal bone loss, focusing on common inflammatory pathways and related changes in bone and calcium metabolism.

K. Gastric Ulcers

Periodontal disease, periodontal bone loss, and tooth loss are associated with gastric ulcers. Investigators have found that the ulcer-causing bacterium, Helicobacter pylori (H. pylori), is much more common in the dental plaque of patients with gastric (peptic) ulcers than in those without ulcers. H. pylori, associated with both stomach ulcers and stomach cancer, "was significantly more common in the stomachs of patients with gum disease than in those without the condition." (Cowen). H. pylori is found in the deeper pockets associated with periodontal disease and in the stomachs of patients with gastric ulcers. Infection from the oral cavity appears to be a causative factor, and gastric ulcer treatment should include treatment of any periodontal disease present.

L. Arthritis

Patients with rheumatoid arthritis (RA) have eight times the incidence of periodontitis compared to non-RA patients. Periodontitis and RA are both inflammatory diseases, sharing common inflammatory pathways. Treatment of the infection and inflammation of periodontal disease improved the signs and symptoms of RA, as reported in a recent study by Case Western University and University Hospitals of Cleveland. Older studies had shown that antibiotics given to treat the RA improved the arthritis condition, but actually treated the periodontitis.

Both RA and periodontitis inflammatory pathways involve Tumor Necrosis Factor-alpha (TNF-alpha) and when RA/periodontitis patients were treated with periodontal tooth-scaling therapy and/or anti-TNF-alpha drug therapy, improvement in RA symptoms was seen in those patients receiving periodontal therapy and in those receiving the drug; greatest improvement occurred in those patients receiving both. Control of periodontitis-associated inflammatory mediators, by either means, improved the RA.

Non-smokers with moderate-to-severe gum disease have nine times the incidence of RA compared to non-periodontitis controls and those with periodontitis have higher blood levels of an antibody associated with more severe RA. Antibodies to P.gingivalis, a periodontitis-involved bacteria, cross-react to chemical mediators (citrullinated proteins) of rheumatoid arthritis.

Inflammation from periodontitis and from RA share common pathways and common factors. Increase in one aggravates the other; treatment of one improves outcomes in the other.

M. Obstructive Sleep Apnea (OSA) and Sleep Disordered Breathing (SDB)

Obstructive Sleep Apnea, which is treatable with C-PAP and/or dental appliances, can cause or worsen excessive daytime sleepiness, obesity, diabetes, hypertension, stroke, kidney disease, misdiagnosed "ADHD," bruxism (excessive tooth grinding), headaches and marital disharmony. OSA and SDB are increased with use of alcohol, benzodiazepines, opioids, and Viagra.

Though C-PAP is highly effective, dental sleep appliances have greater compliance and are indicated in those patients intolerant of C-PAP. OSA and SDB cause changes in chemical, oxidative, and hormonal pathways, initiating and worsening many cardiovascular diseases, hypertension, cardiac arrhythmias (especially atrial fibrillation), MI, stroke, heart failure and atherosclerosis. OSA causes repetitive hypoxias with sympathetic stimulation of the carotid bodies and resultant hypertension. Dementia is often a function of OSA.

OSA and SDB are also causative factors in obesity, diabetes type II, increased risk of gestational hypertension, and gestational diabetes. Increased gestational blood pressure, often with no snoring, can lead to fetal agitation. Pregnancy with snoring is often predictive of gestational hypertension. Untreated severe obstructive sleep apnea doubles the 12-year mortality rate in the general population. Newly developed atrial fibrilation is often a function of obstructive sleep apnea.

Anti-depressants cause sedation in one third of patients, and many of these patients are OSA patients. These OSA patients, successfully treated with CPAP or Oral Sleep Appliances, may still be sleepy as a result of taking their anti-depressants.

N. Snoring and Sleep Disordered Breathing (SDB)

Snoring (even "benign" snoring) vibrations have been shown to cause neural damage in the upper airway neurons and muscles, causing decreased airway neuro-muscular reflex, decreased dilator muscle function (not totally reversible, even with treatment), impaired dilation reflex and upper airway collapse during sleep.

Snoring can, therefore, cause progressive obstructive sleep apnea with the damage not reversible, even with treatment. Early snoring and apnea treatment can lessen future apnea and sleep-disordered breathing problems.

Down's Syndrome patients experience a high (50-80%) rate of sleep-disordered breathing problems.

Pediatric tonsil/adenoid problems and snoring are diagnostic of SDB and predictive of future Obstructive Sleep Apnea.

O. Gastro-Esophageal Reflux Disease (GERD)

Gastro-Esophageal Reflux Disease can cause rapid destruction of the teeth as well as severe metabolic and physiologic problems. Solving this problem from the medical, dental and emotional standpoints is critical for the long-term health and well-being of our patients. (See Section R on Dental Erosion, p.229)

P. Headaches And Temporomandibular Disorders ("TMD" or "TMJ")

Headaches and facial pain are often the result of clenching, grinding, and bite imbalances. Treatment of "TMD" or "TMJ" can help resolve migraines, tension headaches, neurological problems, equilibrium issues, facial pain and associated psychological/emotional problems.

Nocturnal bruxism (often with headaches, facial pain and jaw pain) is associated with Obstructive Sleep Apnea and evidence indicates it may be the result of CNS-activation of jaw and airway dilator muscles to open the airway.

Q. Oral Ulcers: Recurrent Apthous Ulcers (RAU) and Burning Mouth Syndrome (BMS)

Recurrent Apthous Ulcers (RAU) and Burning Mouth Syndrome (BMS) may be the result of many factors, including food sensitivities, chemical (toothpaste, mouthrinse) sensitivities, vitamin/mineral deficiencies, drug reactions, and metabolic changes. RAU share many common causes with burning mouth syndrome and burning tongue syndrome; proper diagnosis can result in appropriate, not merely palliative, treatment.

R. Dental Erosion and Systemic Factors

Dental erosion is loss of tooth structure caused by chemical (usually acid) solutions dissolving tooth structure. The erosion can occur on any or all of the teeth and be the result of intrinsic (body-produced) or extrinsic (food or drink) acid attack. Severe dental changes can result in bite collapse, dental disfiguration, and oral destruction. Intrinsic acid attack may be the result of G.E.R.D., nausea, vomiting from gastro-intestinal and metabolic disturbances; also diseases of the stomach, intestines, pancreas and liver, as well as pregnancy and dysmenorrhea. Gastritis and sinusitis can trigger gagging, vomiting, and G.E.R.D. Many gastro-intestinal, neurological, metabolic, endocrine, and Ob/Gyn disorders can trigger gastric acid reflux. Psychological disorders such as anorexia and bulimia can trigger voluntary or involuntary release of stomach acids into the mouth, as can side-effects of many medications. Many medications such as anti-psychotics, tranquilizers, muscle relaxants, anti-anxiety medications, anti-depressants, and acid-reducers can cause severely decreased salivation (dry-mouth) so that there is not enough saliva to wash away and buffer oral acids; decay and erosion then become rampant.

Sodas, energy drinks, sports drinks, flavored waters, and drinks for metabolite replacement/rehydration (recommended for sports activities, Crohn's Disease, and other metabolic disorders) are usually highly acidic and tooth-destructive. These drinks must be used sparingly, carefully, and with specific protective protocols, which we can provide. Toothbrushing should always be avoided immediately after oral acid exposure to protect temporarily weakened enamel.

It is important to note that careful dental sleuthing can often define the oral pattern (position, surfaces, speed, path and type) of chemical erosion, and determine the origin and cause. Often, diagnosis requires accurate dental models to differentiate erosion vs. bruxism/wear vs. erosion with wear vs. toothbrush abrasion vs. abfractions ("stress corrosion") vs. combination etiologies. We can then refer for proper medical management and provide protective protocols. Definitive dental treatment is usually postponed until the problems are under medical and psychological control.

S. Xerostomia (Dry Mouth) with Dental Decay and Erosion

Xerostomia (dry mouth, decreased salivation) can be the result of age, primary or secondary Sjogren's Disease, rheumatoid problems, and many metabolic/systemic disorders. Many of the current medications for anxiety, sleep, G.E.R.D., muscle problems, hypertension, stress, depression and ADHD can cause decreased salivation and dry-mouth.

The use of multiple medications almost guarantees that many of our patients on medications will experience xerostomia. (Medication change can often reduce the problem severity.) Dry mouth indicates lack of saliva, so there is not enough saliva to wash away or buffer the intrinsic, extrinsic or bacterial acids attacking the teeth. Severe tooth erosion and decay can result, and be aggravated by the use of hard, acidic candies for the dry mouth. This destruction can occur with a 40% loss of salivation; the patient may not notice or report a dry mouth until there is a 70% or greater loss of salivation. We can diagnose xerostomia, recommend oral-protective protocols, and refer back for medical and pharmacological consult.

T. Denture Problems

Ill-fitting and worn dentures can cause bite collapse. Malnutrition can result from decreased protein consumption with increased carbohydrate intake. The loss of jaw and bite support can result in temporomandibular joint ("TMJ") problems and muscle dysfunction with subsequent oral pain, facial pain and headache. Worn dentures can also result in decreased esthetics, patient embarrassment, unwillingness to socialize, isolation, and decreased quality of life. Dementia appears to be aggravated by a bad bite (especially with bad dentures) and the resultant improper brain function. Properly made dentures, often combined with implants, can greatly improve one's outlook, quality of life, and function.

Suggested Additional Readings

My thanks to Dr. Lee Ostler, Jr. All links were active at time of printing.

CONNECTION BETWEEN PERIODONTITIS & C-REACTIVE PROTEIN (CRP):

Inflammation, C-Reactive Protein, and Atherothrombosis. [... There is abundant clinical evidence demonstrating that many biomarkers of inflammation are elevated years in advance of first ever myocardial infarction (MI) or thrombotic stroke and that these same biomarkers are highly predictive of recurrent MI, recurrent stroke, diabetes, and cardiovascular death. In daily practice, the inflammatory biomarker in widest use is high-sensitivity C-reactive protein (hsCRP).... This article ... offers the possibility that other disorders characterized by inflammation, such as periodontal disease, may have an indirect role by influencing the risk, manifestation, and progression of vascular events.] Ridker, P.M., Silvertown, J.D. *Journal of Periodontology* (2008, August), 79(8s), 1544-1551. http://www.joponline.org/doi/full/10.1902/jop.2008.080249

PERIODONTITIS & CARDIAC DISEASE:

Angiographically confirmed coronary heart disease and periodontal disease in middle-aged males. [There was an association between coronary heart disease and poor periodontal status in the middle-aged males investigated. This association was independent of diabetes and all other cardiovascular risk factors investigated.] Briggs, J.E., McKeown, P.P., et al. *Journal of Periodontology*, (2006, January), 77(1), 95-102. doi:10.1902/jop.2006.77.1.95
http://www.joponline.org/doi/abs/10.1902/jop.2006.77.1.95?prevSearch=keywordsfield%3AC- reactive_protein

Cardiovascular disease and the role of oral bacteria. [...Over the decades our understanding of the pathogenesis of CVD has increased, and infections, including those caused by oral bacteria, are more likely involved in CVD progression than previously thought. While many studies have now shown an association between periodontal disease and CVD, the mechanisms underpinning this relationship remain unclear. This review gives a brief overview of the host-bacterial interactions in periodontal disease and virulence factors of oral bacteria before discussing the proposed mechanisms by which oral bacterial may facilitate the progression of CVD.] Leishman, S.J., Do, H.L., et al. *Journal of Oral Microbiology* (2010, December), 2, 5781. doi:10.3402/jom.v2i0.5781
http://www.journaloforalmicrobiology.net/index.php/jom/article/view/5781/6549

Markers of systemic bacterial exposure in periodontal disease and cardiovascular disease risk: A systematic review and meta-analysis. [...Periodontal disease with elevated bacterial exposure is associated with CHD events and early atherogenesis (CIMT), suggesting that the level of systemic bacterial exposure from periodontitis is the biologically pertinent exposure with regard to atherosclerotic risk.] Mustapha, I.Z., Debrey, S., et al. *Journal of Periodontology* (2007 December), 78(12), 2289-2302. http://www.joponline.org/doi/abs/10.1902/jop.2007.070140

PERIODONTITIS & STROKE:

The association between cumulative periodontal disease and stroke history in older adults. [Based on the results of this study, there is evidence of an association between cumulative periodontal disease, based on PHS, and a history of stroke. However, it is unclear whether cumulative periodontal disease is an independent risk factor for stroke or a risk marker for the disease.] Lee, H.J., Garcia, R.I., Journal of Periodontology (2006, October), 77(10), 1744-1754. doi:10.1902/jop.2006.050339 http://www.joponline.org/doi/abs/10.1902/jop.2006.050339?journalCode=jop

PERIODONTITIS & PREGNANCY:

Periodontal diseases and health: Consensus report of the sixth European workshop on periodontology. [... Adverse pregnancy outcome: The findings indicate a likely association between periodontal disease and an increased risk of adverse pregnancy outcomes. ...The impact of periodontal therapy must be further investigated.] Kinane, D., Bouchard, P., et al. *Journal of Clinical Periodontology* (2008, September), 35(s8), 333-337.
http://onlinelibrary.wiley.com/doi/10.1111/j.1600-051X.2008.01278.x/abstract

***Fusobacterium nucleatum* induces premature and term stillbirths in pregnant mice: Implication of oral bacteria in preterm birth.** [*Fusobacterium nucleatum* is a gram-negative anaerobe ubiquitous to the oral cavity. It is associated with periodontal disease. It is also associated with preterm birth and has been isolated from the amniotic fluid, placenta, and chorioamnionic membranes of women delivering prematurely. Periodontal disease is a newly recognized risk factor for preterm birth. This study examined the possible mechanism underlying the link between these two diseases. ...This study represents the first evidence that F. nucleatum may be transmitted hematogenously to the placenta and cause adverse pregnancy outcomes. The results strengthen the link between periodontal disease and preterm birth. Our study also indicates that invasion may be an important virulence mechanism for F. nucleatum to infect the placenta.] Han, Y.W., Redline, R.W., et al. *Infection and Immunity* (2004, April), 72(4), 2272– 2279. doi:10.1128/IAI.72.4.2272-2279.2004
http://www.ncbi.nlm.nih.gov/pmc/articles/PMC375172/

Intrauterine growth restriction, low birth weight, and preterm birth: Adverse pregnancy outcomes and their association with maternal periodontitis. [It has been suggested that periodontitis is associated with systemic alterations such as adverse pregnancy outcomes. However, some conflicting results have been reported. This case-control study was conducted to determine the association between maternal periodontitis and preterm birth (PTB), low birth weight (LBW), and intrauterine growth restriction (IUGR)...Results emphasize the importance of periodontal care in prenatal health programs.] Siqueira, F.M., Cota, L.O.M., Costa, J.E. *Journal of Periodontology* (2007, December), 78(12), 2266-2276. http://www.joponline.org/doi/abs/10.1902/jop.2007.070196

Periodontal therapy may reduce the risk of preterm low birth weight in women with periodontal disease: A randomized controlled trial. [Pregnant women who receive treatment for their periodontal disease can reduce their risk of giving birth to a low birth-weight or pre- term baby. ...] Lopez, N.J., et al. *Journal of Periodontology* (2002, August), 73(8) 911-924. http://www.joponline.org/doi/abs/10.1902/jop.2002.73.8.911

OBESITY & DIABETES:

Association of periodontal parameters with metabolic level, systemic inflammatory markers in type 2 diabetes patients. [Backgrounds: While world-wide evidence tends to prove that diabetes adversely affects periodontal health, there is insufficient clue that periodontitis may aggravate metabolic controlling and systemic inflammation. This study... aims to clarify the relationship of periodontal parameters with metabolic level as well as systemic inflammatory markers in diabetes patients. ...] Chen, L., Wei, B., et al. *Journal of Periodontology* (2010, March), 81(3), 364-371. doi:10.1902/jop.2009.090544
http://www.joponline.org/doi/abs/10.1902/jop.2009.090544?journalCode=jop

Clinical and metabolic changes after conventional treatment of type 2 diabetic patients with chronic periodontitis. [The aim of this study was to compare the response to conventional periodontal treatment between patients with or without type 2 diabetes mellitus from a clinical and metabolic standpoint. ...] Faria-Almeida, R., Navarro, A., et al. *Journal of Periodontology* (2006, April), 77(4), 591-598. doi: 10.1902/jop.2006.050084
http://www.joponline.org/doi/abs/10.1902/jop.2006.050084

Obesity and periodontal disease in young, middle-aged, and older adults. [Background: The growing prevalence of increased body weight and obesity in the United States has raised significant public health concerns. ... Conclusions: In a younger population, overall and abdominal obesity are associated with increased prevalence of periodontal disease, while underweight (BMI <18.5) is associated with decreased prevalence...] Al-Zahrani, M.S., Bissada, N.F., et al. *Journal of Periodontology* (2003, May), 74, 610-615. http://www.joponline.org/doi/abs/10.1902/jop.2003.74.5.610

KIDNEY DISEASE:
Clinical and serologic markers of periodontal infection and chronic kidney disease. [Background: Chronic kidney disease and its concomitant sequelae represent a major public health problem. Recent data suggest periodontal infection contributes to chronic kidney disease. Methods: This United States population–based study of 4,053 adults ≥40 years of age investigated the association between chronic kidney disease and clinical measures and serologic markers of periodontal infection. ...] Fisher, M.A., Taylor, G.W., et al. *Journal of Periodontology* (2008, September), 79(9), 1670-1678. http://www.joponline.org/doi/abs/10.1902/jop.2008.070569

RESPIRATORY PROBLEMS & LUNG DISEASE
Involvement of periodontopathic anaerobes in aspiration pneumonia. [Increasing evidence has linked the anaerobic bacteria forming periodontopathic biofilms with aspiration pneumonia in elderly persons.] Okuda, K. et al. *Journal of Periodontology* (2005, November), 76(11-s), 2154-2160.
http://www.joponline.org/doi/abs/10.1902/jop.2005.76.11-S.2154

OSTEOPOROSIS:
Periodontal diseases and osteoporosis: Association and mechanisms. [There is increasing evidence that osteoporosis, and the underlying loss of bone mass characteristic of this disease, is associated with periodontal disease and tooth loss. ... Current evidence including several prospective studies supports an association of osteoporosis with the onset and progression of periodontal disease in humans. ... Both periodontal disease and osteoporosis are serious public-health concerns in the United States. ... This paper reviews the current evidence on the association between periodontal disease and osteoporosis.] Wactawski-Wende, J. *Annals of Periodontology* (2001, December), 6(1), 197-208.
http://www.joponline.org/doi/abs/10.1902/annals.2001.6.1.197

The relationship between bone mineral density and periodontitis in postmenopausal women. [Skeletal BMD is related to interproximal alveolar bone loss and, to a lesser extent, to clinical attachment loss, implicating postmenopausal osteopenia as a risk indicator for periodontal disease.] Tezal, M., Grossi, S.G., et al. *Journal of Periodontology* (2000, September), 71(9), 1492-1498.
http://www.joponline.org/doi/abs/10.1902/jop.2000.71.9.1492

GASTRIC ULCERS:
Are dental plaque, poor oral hygiene, and periodontal disease associated with *Helicobacter pylori* infection? [The microorganism Helicobacter pylori has been closely linked to chronic gastritis, peptic ulcer, gastric cancer, and mucosa-associated lymphoid tissue (MALT) lymphoma. Despite the current treatment regimens that lead to successful management of H. pylori-positive chronic gastritis, the reinfection rate is high. ...] Anand, P.S., Nandakumar, K. *Journal of Periodontology* (2006, April), 77(4), 692-698. http://www.joponline.org/doi/abs/10.1902/jop.2006.050163

ARTHRITIS:
Is there a relationship between rheumatoid arthritis and periodontal disease? [Because of several similar features in the pathobiology of periodontitis and rheumatoid arthritis, in a previous study we proposed a possible **relationship** between the two diseases. ... **Conclusions:** The results of this study provide further evidence of a significant association between periodontitis and rheumatoid arthritis. ...] Mercado, F., Marshall, R.I., et al. *Journal of Clinical Periodontology* (2011, June), 72(6) 779-787.
http://www.blackwell-synergy.com/doi/abs/10.1034/j.1600- 051x.2000.027004267.x?journalCode=cpe

TEMPOROMANDIBULAR PROBLEMS:
Inflammatory cytokines activity in temporomandibular joint disorders: a review of literature. [Cytokines are important polypeptides mediators of acute and chronic inflammation. These molecules act as a complex immunological network, ... In spite of some controversial findings, in general high levels of pro-inflammatory cytokines have been correlated with signs and symptoms of temporomandibular disorders (TMD) such as internal derangement and osteoarthritis. These mediators promote degradation of cartilage and bone joint by inducing release of proteinases and other inflammatory molecules...]. Campos, M.I.G., Campos, P.S.F., et al. *Brazilian Journal of Oral Sciences* (2006, July-September), 5(18).
http://www.fop.unicamp.br/brjorals/temp2/c18_Art1_inflammatory.pdf

DENTAL EROSION & SYSTEMIC FACTORS
HIV Infection and Bone Loss Due to Periodontal Disease [Purpose: The goal of this study was to determine whether HIV infection and/or high-risk behaviors associated with HIV infection are related to alveolar bone loss in a sample of subjects screened at a dental school clinic. ... Conclusion: These results suggest that HIV infection is not related to alveolar bone loss in individuals with high risk behaviors for HIV infection. These results also suggest that previously reported relationships between HIV infection and increased alveolar bone loss may be explained by other factors, such as smoking. Individuals in this study population with risk behaviors associated with HIV infection, smoked at a high rate, and due to the smoking behavior have a high rate of periodontal disease.] Aichelmann-Reidy, M.E., Wrigley, D., et al. *Journal of Periodontology* (2010, June), 81(6), 877-884. http://www.joponline.org/doi/abs/10.1902/jop.2010.070675

XEROSTOMIA WITH DENTAL DECAY & EROSION
Using Probiotics to help patients be proactive: Novel approach can enable the prevention of root caries in a periodontal geriatric population. [As the US population ages, ...a greater percentage of patients are keeping more teeth. ... [T]eeth retention for a large portion of adults may require some periodontal therapy.... Age- or medication-induced xerostomia diminishes the innate ability of saliva's protective response. Root surfaces are uniquely more susceptible to caries as they are more porous and likely to develop biofilms and, ultimately, dental caries. ... Recently, a new oral probiotic entered the marketplace that can uniquely help prevent root surface decay. By continually inoculating the oral cavity with probiotic bacteria that out-compete naturally occurring S. mutans, an environment is created that combats the development of dental caries.] Oxford, G.E. *Inside Dentistry* (2011, March), 7(3), 96-100. http://editiondigital.net/publication/?i=61413

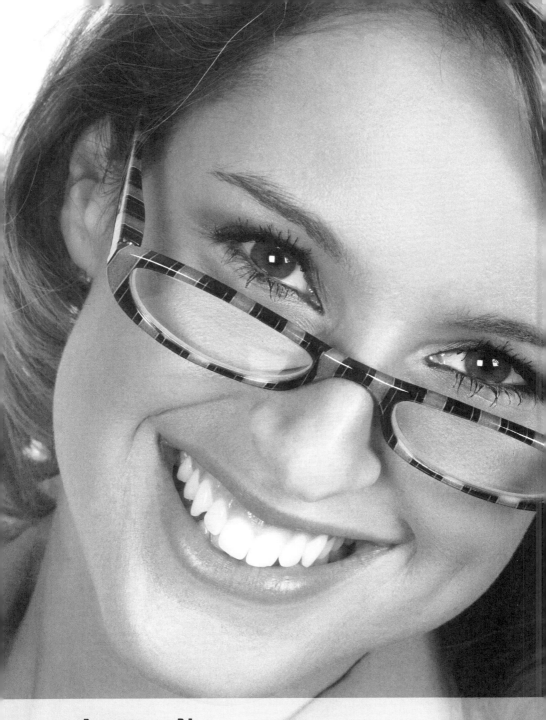

Appendix:
Instructions for Patients

Treatment of Chronic Bad Breath

Recommendations:

1. Evaluation by your dentist for oral infections

2. Evaluation by your dentist for other oral-odor-causing conditions

3. Evaluation of your diet for odor-causing foods

4. Possible evaluation by your physician for any medical or systemic factors affecting your breath

5. If systemic factors and oral infections are eliminated as causes of your bad breath, use flossing, brushing, tongue scraping and oral rinses (as indicated) for treatment

Tooth Whitening

Thank you for giving us the opportunity to brighten your smile. Hopefully, this will be an exciting time for you.

The more you bleach consistently, the more quickly you will see the results, but the key is comfort, not speed!

After we have delivered your bleaching trays, you will need to return to our office when you have almost completed the gel provided.

Please bring your trays to each visit!!!

Homecare:

1. Always brush and floss after using the gel and trays; never immediately before.
2. Brushing and flossing may be done two hours prior to bleaching. (sooner if comfortable)
3. We recommend that you use a desensitizing toothpaste with a high level of fluoride protection. We have included Fluoridex with your bleaching kit.
4. Never use a tartar-control toothpaste!
5. Rinse trays under cold water; never under hot or warm water!

Directions:

1. Wear trays nightly for approximately 5-8 hours; if sensitive, see below.
2. Fill the trays ¼ full (=one "drop") in the front eight to ten teeth; including bicuspids; no molars.
3. Do not fill the molar teeth area with gel.
4. Spit out excess gel (should be minimal).
5. Wipe away excess gel with fingers. If too much excess; use less gel next time.
6. DO NOT RINSE YOUR MOUTH WITH FILLED TRAYS IN PLACE.

7. Upon waking, rinse trays in cold water, never in warm or hot water.
8. Store in a dry, safe place.
9. Brush and floss as usual.

If sensitivity occurs:

1. Decrease the length of time that you wear the trays at night; two hours provides 90% of the whitening.
2. Use the trays and gel every other night,
3. Apply Fluoridex or fluoride gel in the tray every other night instead of the bleaching gel, using an irrigating syringe to place one drop in each tooth location in the tray.
4. Call our office and let us know about the sensitivity.

Please be aware:

1. Some characteristics of the teeth may become more noticeable with tooth brightening. These include cracks, craze lines, "white spots"' hypo/hyper-calcifications, etc. These are natural components of esthetics and are not caused by the brightening process.
2. Pet Owners: Cats and dogs love the smell of the trays and will chew on them if left in their reach or on an open counter-top.

Avoid:

- Syringes of gel getting hot/warm (will inactivate)
- Trays becoming warm/ hot (will distort)
- Eating or drinking with trays in place
- Chewing food with trays in place (will break trays)
- Drinking hot or colored liquids with trays in place (will distort/ stain trays)
- Tartar- Control Toothpaste (will make teeth sensitive)
- Leaving trays in reach of pets (they will get eaten!)

Please remember that no dental treatment can be done until three-four weeks after bleaching is completed.

Care of Your New Dental Restorations (fillings)

We have just placed dental restorations (fillings) in your teeth and these should serve you for many years. If the fillings are large, you may have been told that a crown may be needed in the future. You should be aware of the following information, so your fillings will serve as long as possible.

Strength and chewing:

Dental restorations continue to get stronger over the first 24 hours. Please do not chew on your new fillings for 24 hours; liquid and totally soft foods are best. Do not attempt to chew hard foods on the "other" side as you can easily forget and over-stress the new fillings, causing a crack or failure that may not become evident for days, weeks, or years. Remember, always, that chewing on hard foods, like nuts, bones, corn nuts, and ice, can break teeth, so they should be avoided in the future.

Sensitivity:

Teeth with new fillings are often sensitive to hot and cold. This sensitivity should settle down over the next few days; if it does not, please contact us. As the bite "settles in," too hard a bite on the new fillings can cause sensitivity. Please inform us of any sensitivity or bite problems. Please use only toothpaste with a high level of fluoride for desensitization and protection. We can provide you with Fluoridex. Avoid toothpastes with tartar control, baking soda and whitening.

Recalls:

Please visit us at regular three-month or six-months recall periods. Often, problems that are developing around the restorations can be found at an early stage and corrected easily. Waiting longer may require re-doing the entire restoration or a larger restorative procedure.

Preventative procedures after fillings:

Use the following procedures to protect your teeth:

a. Brush twice daily; brush and floss at bedtime.

b. Use high-level fluoride toothpaste (from us or by prescription) and possibly a fluoride rinse.

Avoid hard foods and acidic drinks (sodas, energy drinks, sports drinks, etc).

The Future:

Small silver amalgams and composite restorations should serve for many years in your mouth. However, large restorations may break or the tooth structure around them may break in the future. In this event, the involved tooth or teeth will require a crown (cap) for optimum strength.

Problems:

If any of the following problems occur, contact us immediately to avoid further problems:

a. A feeling of movement or looseness in the restoration or tooth

b. Sensitivity to sweet foods, cold, biting, or chewing

c. A peculiar taste from the restoration site.

d. Breakage of a piece of material from the restoration

e. Breakage of tooth structure

We have done our best to provide you with the finest quality oral restorations available today.

However, as with a fine automobile or watch, only your continuous care and concern can assure optimum service and longevity.

Homecare for Daily Wear Appliance

1. Wear appliance daily.

2. Take out every night.

3. Brush the appliance with a soft toothbrush with water, liquid soap, or mouthwash (no toothpaste). Every two or three days, let it soak in a denture bath with one denture cleaning tablet for 20 minutes (while washing, showering or dressing). If your appliance has metal parts, use a denture soak that is "Safe for Metal" or "Safe for Partials."

4. Remove from denture bath, rinse and store in clear cool water.

5. Never clean the appliance in the washing machine, dryer, dishwasher or in hot water. Do not store in a hot car.

6. Please keep this (and all other oral appliances) away from pets (cats and dogs). Pets love the smell and taste of your oral appliances and will even climb to reach them. These appliances can easily be chewed up and destroyed by the pet.

7. Please inform us immediately if any adjustments are needed or if anything prevents wear of the appliance. Lack of wear (for any reason), even for a short time, will allow normal shifting of the teeth. You may then not be able to wear the appliance and your investment may be wasted.

Homecare for Night Wear Appliance
(retainers, nightguards, sleep apnea appliances)

1. Place the appliance in at night when going to sleep. Place fluoride gel in appliance (sparingly; one small drop per tooth).

2. Remove the appliance every morning.

3. Brush the appliance with a soft toothbrush with water, liquid soap or mouthwash (no toothpaste). Every two or three days, let it soak in a denture bath with one denture cleaning tablet for 20 minutes (while washing, showering or dressing). If your appliance has metal parts, use a denture soak that is "Safe for Metal" or "Safe for Partials."

4. Remove it from the denture bath, rinse, and store in clear cool water during the day.

5. Never clean the appliance in the washing machine, dryer, dishwasher or in hot water. Do not store in a hot car.

6. Please keep this (and all other oral appliances) away from pets (cats and dogs). Pets love the smell and taste of your oral appliances and will even climb to reach them. These appliances can easily be chewed up and destroyed by the pet.

7. Please inform us immediately if any adjustments are needed or if anything prevents wear of the appliance. Lack of wear (for any reason), even for a short time, will allow normal shifting of the teeth. You may then not be able to wear the appliance and your investment may be wasted.

Post-Operative Instructions for Oral Surgery

Extractions and bone grafts

1. Bleeding will likely be present for several hours, and oozing which results in bright red saliva is common for 24 hours after surgery. Bite gently on gauze for two hours after your surgery. This allows a clot to form, insuring proper healing. Fresh gauze (which we have given you) may be inserted every hour. Should bleeding continue after two hours, bite gently on a wet tea bag for one-two hours using a standard, non-herbal, tea bag. Avoid rinsing for 24 hours, and call us if your mouth fills with large blood clots.

2. Swelling is to be expected, often peaks on the third day, and is usually gone by the seventh day. Apply an ice bag to the side of your face where the surgery was performed to help reduce the swelling. Hold ice in place for 20 minutes on and 20 minutes off for 48 hours. Some swelling and discoloration of the skin are common and need not cause alarm. However, if swelling continues to enlarge after three days or if the swelling is hot/red, contact our office immediately. Normal swelling may last for seven to ten days. Sleeping with the head elevated (an extra pillow or two) can help reduce swelling and discomfort. Starting three days after surgery (two days of using ice + one extra day), moist heat (heating pad, microwaved heating pad with cover, or hot water bottle) will help reduce residual swelling.

3. Food: Please do not eat, drink, or rinse your mouth for three hours after surgery except to take medication. After three hours, begin with liquid foods for seven days and then soft/liquid foods for three weeks. Avoid foods likely to get caught in the surgery site or tear the stitches

such as chips, nuts, rice, popcorn, etc. Avoid hot food, hot drinks, or active chewing while your mouth is still numb; avoid very hot food and drinks for two weeks. Blenderized (drinkable) foods, and protein/nutritional drinks are very helpful during this period. Drink at least six-eight large glasses of liquids per day to avoid dehydration, fever, possible shock, and possible hospitalization.

4. Stitches (sutures) may dissolve on their own or may need to be removed in one week. This will be taken care of at your post-operative appointment. Stitches falling out present no problems unless persistent bleeding occurs.

5. Alcohol and smoking should be avoided for three days after extractions and for seven days with grafts.

6. A "dry socket" is more likely to occur if you use alcohol, tobacco (smoking) or birth-control drugs. It usually presents as pain three-seven days after surgery at the extraction site, not relieved by pain medications, and will be treated with placement of a medicated dressing.

7. Avoid the following during the recuperation period:

    - Spitting or rinsing hard for several days
    - Using a straw
    - Carbonated (fizzy) drinks
    - Smoking for three days for extractions and one week for grafts
    - Alcohol for three days for extractions and one week for grafts
    - Sedatives
    - Hot liquids
    - Electric toothbrush or vigorous toothbrushing
    - Vigorous activity for 48 hours
    - Contact sports for one week.

8. Oral Hygiene will speed healing and reduce odor and infection: One day after surgery, begin rinsing your mouth gently with warm (not hot) salt water (one rounded teaspoon of salt in a tall glass of warm water.). Allow the salty water to remain in the mouth for 30 seconds. DO NOT rinse vigorously. Rinse four times daily for five days. You may also begin brushing and flossing all your teeth to remove plaque. Please use a fluoride toothpaste. Over-the-counter mouth rinses may be used if diluted in half with water.

9. Discomfort and Pain Medications: Follow directions on the bottle. Expect two-three days of possible discomfort following removal of impacted teeth. Take over-the-counter ibuprophen (Motrin, Advil, Nuprin), naproxyn (Naprosyn, Aleve), aspirin or Tylenol regularly for three-five days as recommended. Add in your prescription pain medication as needed. Take your medication before the numbness wears off.

    Begin taking your pain medication soon enough that it has time to take effect prior to the numbing medicine wearing off. Pain medication can cause an upset stomach and nausea, therefore, it is best to take it with food. Any medication which may cause stomach upset and nausea should be taken with a tall hot/warm drink, soft foods and/or antacids. (Ask your Pharmacist.) You should rest (minimize movement) when taking narcotic pain medications and call us if vomiting occurs.

    Begin your antibiotic medication right away, then continue to follow the directions on the bottle.

    Begin the Peridex Rinse tomorrow and continue to rinse for 30 seconds twice daily for two weeks

10. Fever (under 101°) is usually due to decreased fluid intake, vomiting and dehydration. It usually responds well to increased fluid intake (at least six-eight large glasses of liquid per day). Fever of 102° and above may be a sign of infection, and you should notify us immediately.

11. Please call us if you experience any of the following:

   • Vomiting
   • Generalized rash or itch
   • Bloody or persistent diarrhea
   • Increasing pain or swelling after the third day
   • Fever greater than 101°
   • Foul taste or discharge in the mouth
   • Numbness continuing for more than twelve hours
   • Other surgery-related problems

Post-Operative Instructions for Extraction with Sinus Involvement

1. Please do not sneeze or blow through your nose for two weeks. If you need to sneeze, sneeze through your mouth.

2. Claritin – D-24 hr or Zyrtec – D-24 hr: one tablet one time per day for two weeks.

3. Amoxicillin 500 mg – three times a daily or 875 mg twice daily for two weeks (or other antibiotic if penicillin-allergic).

4. Long acting nasal spray twice daily for five days.

5. Take pain and other medication as directed (on the bottle).

6. Bite firmly on gauze for two hours after your surgery. This allows a clot to form, insuring proper healing. Should bleeding continue after two hours, bite gently on a wet tea bag for one hour, using a standard (non-herbal) tea bag.

7. Apply an ice bag to the side of your face where the surgery was done to help reduce swelling. Ice should be held in place for 24/48 hours (20 minutes on and 20 minutes off).

8. Please do not eat, drink or rinse your mouth for three hours and do not rinse or spit hard for one day. It is important not to disturb the clot until it is fully formed.

   After three hours and for one day, drink what you want, except for alcohol and hot beverages in small gentle sips on the other side of your mouth. Do not rinse or swish.

   If you need to spit, do so very gently.

9. One day after surgery, begin rinsing your mouth gently with warm (not hot) salt water (tall glass of warm water with a rounded teaspoon of salt). Allow salty water to remain in the mouth for thirty (30) seconds. DO NOT rinse vigorously. Please rinse four times a day for five days.

10. If you had stitches put in your mouth, you may need to come back to the office in one week to have them removed and healing checked.

11. You should eat soft foods for a few days because your gums will be sore. Begin eating regular foods when it is comfortable for you. Smoking should be avoided for one week to minimize possible complications. Drink at least six-eight large glasses of liquid per day to avoid dehydration and fever.

12. Some swelling and discoloration of the skin are common and need not cause alarm.

    If you have excessive bleeding, pain, fever or other severe problems, contact our office immediately.

Post-Operative Instructions for Periodontal (Gum) Surgery & Periodontal (Gum) Grafts

1. Bleeding will likely be present for several hours, and oozing which results in bright red saliva is common for 24 hours after surgery. If there is excessive bleeding, remove any clots with a gauze square, and place moderate but constant pressure over the bleeding area with a damp tea bag. Hold in place for at least 30 minutes. If this is not successful, call us. Avoid forceful rinsing for 48 hours; for minor bleeding, gently rinse with cold tea.

2. For Grafts: The (upper) surgical stent should be worn full-time (even while rinsing with water or oral rinse) for three to four days. It may be removed to be washed under cold water and replaced immediately. (Do your rinsing with stent in place.) After four full days, you may wear the stent or not, as comfortable. Leaving it in place will help protect the donor site and reduce bleeding. Always keep your stent available during the first week of healing to put in place should bleeding begin. Bring the stent with you to the office if you need to see us for any bleeding problems.

3. Swelling is to be expected, often peaks on the third day and is usually gone by the seventh day. Apply an ice bag to the side of your face where the surgery was performed to help reduce swelling. Hold ice in place for 20 minutes on and 20 minutes off for 48 hours. Some swelling and discoloration of the skin are common and need not cause alarm. However, if swelling continues to enlarge after three days or if the swelling is hot/red, contact our office immediately. Normal swelling may last for seven-ten days. Sleeping with the head elevated (an extra pillow or two) can help reduce swelling or discomfort. Starting four days after surgery

(two days of using ice + one extra day), moist heat (heating pad, etc.) over the surgerized area will help reduce residual swelling.

4. Food: Please do not eat, drink, or rinse your mouth for three hours after surgery. After three hours, begin with liquid foods for seven days and then soft/ liquid foods for three weeks. Avoid foods likely to get caught in the surgery site or tear the stitches such as chips, nuts, rice, popcorn, etc. Avoid hot food, drinks, or active chewing while your mouth is still numb; avoid very hot food and drinks for two weeks. Blenderized (drinkable) foods, and protein/nutritional drinks are very helpful during this period. Drink at least six-eight large glasses of liquids per day to avoid dehydration, fever, possible shock, and possible hospitalization.

5. Surgical Dressing, if present around your teeth, is to protect the surgical area and facilitate healing. It should stay in place until your next appointment. Small particles of dressing may chip off from time to time; this is normal. If the entire dressing comes loose, or if you feel discomfort, please call. Do not overexercise your mouth or lips or try to see the surgical site. This may accidentally tear the sutures or displace the dressing and graft tissue. Drink cold fluids during the first 24 hours; this will keep the dressing hard.

6. Stitches (sutures) may dissolve on their own or may need to be removed in one week. This will be taken care of at your post-operative appointment. Stitches falling out present no problems unless persistent bleeding occurs or the gum tissue becomes loose.

7. Alcohol and smoking should be avoided for one week following periodontal surgery and gum grafts.

8. Avoid the following during the recuperation period:

   - Spitting or rinsing hard for several days

   - Using a straw

   - Carbonated (fizzy) drinks

   - Smoking and alcohol for one week with periodontal (gum) surgery and grafts

   - Sedatives

   - Hot liquids

   - Electric toothbrush or vigorous tooth brushing

   - Vigorous activity for one week

   - Contact sports for one week or longer

9. Oral Hygiene will speed healing and reduce odor and infection; one day after surgery begin rinsing your mouth gently with warm (not hot) salt water. (one rounded teaspoon of salt in a tall glass of warm water). Allow the salty water to remain in the mouth for 30 seconds but DO NOT rinse vigorously. Rinse four times daily for five days. You may also begin regular brushing and flossing teeth not involved in the surgery. Avoid areas of surgery, sutures, or dressing. Please use fluoride toothpaste. Over-the-counter mouth rinses may be used if diluted in half with water. Your prescription oral rinse should be used for 30 full seconds twice daily.

10. Discomfort and Pain Medications: Follow directions on the bottle. Expect two-three days of significant discomfort following surgery. Take over-the-counter ibprophen (Motrin, Advil, Nuprin), naproxyn (Naprosyn, Aleve), aspirin or Tylenol regularly for three-five days as

recommended. Add in your prescription pain medication as needed. Take your medication before the numbness wears off.

Begin taking your pain medication as directed so that it has time to take effect prior to the numbing wearing off. Pain medication can cause upset stomach and nausea; therefore, it is best to take with food. Any medication which may cause stomach upset and nausea should be taken with a tall, hot/warm drink, soft foods, and/or antacids. (Ask your pharmacist.) You should rest (minimize movement) when taking narcotic pain medications and call us if vomiting occurs.

11. Fever (under 101°) is usually due to decreased fluid intake, vomiting, and dehydration. It usually responds well to increased fluid intake; at least six-eight large glasses of liquid per day. Fever of 102° and above may be a sign of infection and you should notify us immediately.

12. Please call us if you experience any of the following:

- Vomiting

- Generalized rash or itch

- Bloody or persistent diarrhea

- Increasing pain or swelling after the third day

- Fever greater than 101°

- Foul taste or discharge in the mouth

- If numbness continues for more than 12 hours

- Other surgery-related problems

Post-Operative Instructions for Temporary Crowns

We have just placed your temporary crown. A temporary crown should only be worn for three weeks, unless you were told differently by Dr. Finkel.

Discomfort:

1. Your discomfort should be minimal.

2. As necessary for soreness, if not allergic, take ibuprofen (Advil, Nuprin, Motrin) 600 mg with acetaminophen (Tylenol) 1000 mg, together, every six hours with a tall hot drink.

3. You may be given an anti-microbial rinse that should also help with any discomfort to the gum tissue.

Medication:

1. Peridex (Perioguard, etc.) rinse: Rinse ½ oz. for 30 seconds twice daily, after breakfast and before bed. It is very important to use the Peridex rinse until your permanent crown is seated.

2. Should you run out of rinse before your next appointment, please call our office so that we may phone in a refill or have you stop by our office for another bottle at no charge. In some instances, instead of Peridex, we will recommend Oxyfresh or Crest Pro-Health Rinse to be used 30 seconds three times daily.

Should your temporary crown come off:

1. Never eat while your temporary crown is off. Call the office or Dr. Finkel immediately, even if over the weekend.

2. Place Vaseline inside the temporary crown and put it back in place. You may remove the crown for sleep and replace it the next morning.

3. Any delay in replacing the temporary crown may result in the final crown having to be redone at additional cost to you.

Homecare Instructions:

1. Continue to brush as normal, just be gentle around your temporary crown.

2. While flossing, pull the floss straight out sideways from your temporary crown, rather than up and down to remove. We may recommend no flossing, but to use Peridex or other oral rinse, as noted.

3. While using the Peridex rinse, there is no need to floss in the area of your temporary crown. Flossing may dislodge the temporary crown.

Things to avoid while wearing a temporary crown:

1. Hard foods, ice, nuts

2. Sticky foods, chewing gum

3. Coffee, tea and red wine (will stain temporary crowns)

Please Note: ***

If it comes loose, it is very important to have your temporary crown immediately replaced to avoid teeth shifting and gum changes (possibly within one day) which would prevent your final crown from fitting properly. Any delay in replacement of the temporary crown may result in the final crown having to be re-done at additional cost to you.

Post-Operative Instructions for Implant Surgery

This instruction sheet will help you to understand the dental implant placement procedure.

1. Please have a good night's rest before the day of implant placement and eat a nutritious breakfast or lunch (unless having sedation).

2. If sedating, please have not eaten for 10 hours.

3. If sedating, please have taken your night-time medication prior to sleep, on an empty stomach.

4. A local anesthetic will be used to block sensation in the area where the implant is to be placed.

5. A small incision may be made in your gums to obtain access to the location where the implant will be placed.

6. Several sizes of small drills will be used to make precise, painless preparations in the locations where the implants will be placed.

7. Implants will be placed into the prepared sites.

8. Your gum tissue may be sutured together to isolate the newly placed implants from oral fluids and foods. The stitches will dissolve by themselves unless we advise you differently.

9. You will be asked to bite on gauze sponges for at least one half-hour after the implant placement to stabilize any incision and stop any slight blood flow.

10. You will be given at least two prescriptions which you should have filled and begin to use immediately:

    a. An antibiotic to control any potential infection; please take this medication as directed until the tablets are gone. An antimicrobial rinse should be used for 30 seconds, twice daily.

    b. A pain relieving medication to control discomfort. Take this medication only until you do not need it anymore.

11. Anesthesia should remain in your mouth for at least one hour or longer after we are finished.

12. As soon as possible after treatment, place ice in a plastic bag and hold it on the outside of your face for a few hours over the sites where the implants were placed for 20 minutes on and 20 minutes off. This reduces the potential swelling and bruising. However, you may still have some swelling and bruising for a few days.

13. There may be a feeling of numbness caused by the surgery that lingers for a short time. Usually, this feeling goes away within a few days. In a very few cases it does not go away totally.

14. Eat and drink only soft foods for a few days. The less force you put on the implant area for the next several days the better and faster will be the healing. Over 95% of implants are accepted well by the body, and about one out of 20 is rejected and must be replaced.

15. We anticipate that these implants will serve you for many years.

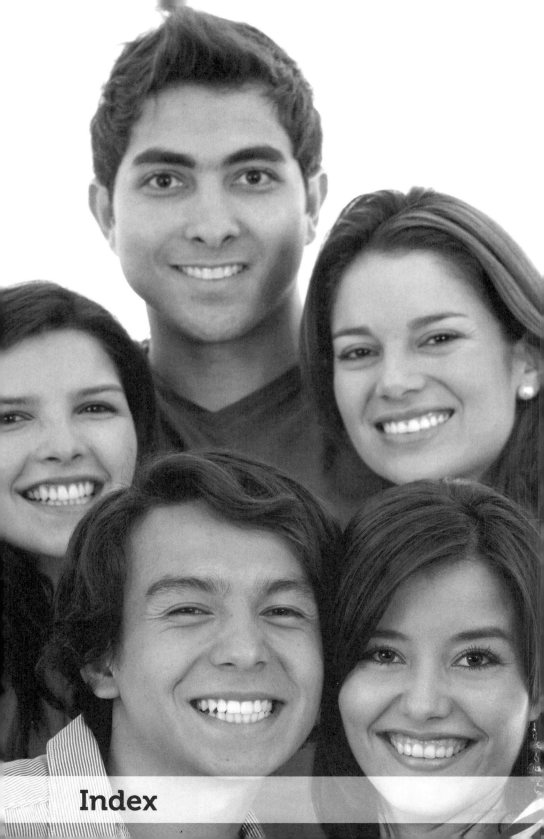

Index

Index

D

E

F

G

P

R

S

T

U

V

W

X

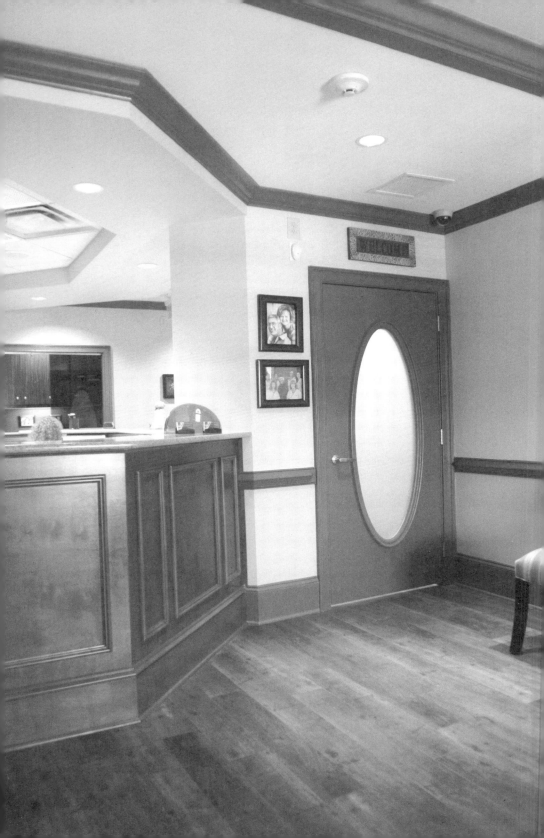